Clinical Electromyography

Clinical Electromyography

J A R LENMAN MB ChB FRCP Ed

Reader in Neurology,
University of Dundee

A E RITCHIE MA BSc MD FRSE

Secretary to the Carnegie Trust
for the Universities of Scotland, Edinburgh

Formerly Professor of Physiology,
University of St Andrews

PHILADELPHIA, TORONTO

J. B. LIPPINCOTT COMPANY

Published in Great Britain in 1970 by
PITMAN MEDICAL & SCIENTIFIC PUBLISHING CO LTD

Published and distributed in North America by
J. B. LIPPINCOTT COMPANY

PRINTED IN GREAT BRITAIN

Contents

Plates

Foreword

The history of electrodiagnosis of paralytic disorders has been a chequered one. The 'electrical reactions' of muscles introduced by Erb (1868) were of little assistance to the clinician, since consistent results were only found in completely denervated muscle with carefully standardised technique. The differential response to galvanic and faradic stimulation of the motor point of muscle is also of little use in detecting partial denervation. Greater discrimination is obtained by plotting an intensity-duration curve using the more accurate electronic stimulators of different types (Ritchie, 1944). Although this method of electrodiagnosis suffers from the more severe practical disadvantages of the earlier methods in being inapplicable to deeply situated muscles and fatiguing to patient and investigator, as it requires detection of threshold contraction responses of muscle, it has the important advantage of being suitable for recording by a technician with limited training. Although quantification of the response by chronaximetry is now of only historical interest, the method is still capable of providing valuable information. Excitability threshold changes in a peripheral nerve may provide diagnostic and prognostic information earlier than any other method of electrodiagnosis. Professor Ritchie has made valuable contributions to the technical and practical aspects of nerve excitability measurement and in this book describes some recent advances that demonstrate its continuing value. If the intensity-duration curve is plotted with a sufficient number of points, inflections ('kinks') indicating a cross-over point from the excitability curve of one unit to another make it possible to detect partial denervation, but this requires a meticulous technique used by few physiotherapists. The fundamental disadvantage of the conventional technique is that it detects the lowest threshold nerve or muscle fibres for each stimulus. It only requires survival of some normal low threshold nerve fibres in a damaged nerve trunk, and the intensity-duration curve will remain normal. The response of higher threshold units can be determined by using an electromyographic index of motor-unit response but the essential simplicity of the method is then lost.

These limitations and the requirements of pheripheral nerve surgery in wartime led to the development of clinical electromyography in the 1940s. Adrian and Bronk's use of the concentric needle electrode in 1929 and the development of differential amplifiers and the cathode-ray oscilloscope had provided the technology for investigating the function of single motor units and their summation in voluntary contractions of different degrees, and, in 1938, Denny-Brown and Pennybacker investigated the spontaneous activity of partially or completely denervated muscle. This technique was exploited by Buchthal and Clemmesen (1941) and Weddell *et al.* (1944) for the investigation of neurogenic muscular atrophy and peripheral nerve injuries.

A new dimension was introduced by Kugelberg (1947) who recognised morphological differences in the motor unit action potentials in muscular disorders. Since then, an important function of electromyography has been the differential diagnosis between neurogenic and myogenic weakness.

In the 1950s interest reverted to the study of peripheral nerve disease and spinal cord function with the introduction of measurement of motor nerve conduction velocity in neuropathies (Simpson, 1956), extended to sensory nerves by Gilliatt and Sears (1958), and the investigation of reflex activity by Magladery and McDougal (1950) and Paillard (1955). Quantitative evaluation of electromyographic data has become essential (Buchthal *et al.*, 1954). Dr Lenman has made valuable contributions on integrated electromyography.

In the present decade the introduction of digital computers for extracting small biogenic signals from 'noise', and for carrying out statistical sorting and cross-correlation procedures, are extending electrodiagnostic techniques and opening the way to detailed quantitative studies of the physiology of the motor unit in health and disease.

These advances have removed electrodiagnosis from the sphere of the medical ancillary, and of the practitioner of physical medicine to that of the clinical neurophysiologist. The time has now come when the vast amount of information must be made available to a generation of physicians and physiologists who have not grown up with it. The physician, usually a neurologist, must have knowledge of the scope and limitations of electrophysical techniques. He must realise that he should ask a physiological question and will receive a physiological answer which he must then integrate with other clinical evidence in making a diagnosis and prognosis. On the other hand, the physiologist must have sufficient training in clinical neurology to understand the nature of the problem and the probable differential diagnosis. In this book the authors have assembled selected data on electrodiagnostic methods. It is not intended to be an exhaustive treatise on clinical neurophysiology, but it provides sufficient neurophysiology for the clinician to understand the nature and scope of the techniques and sufficient clinical information for the physiologist.

The most satisfactory way to learn a technique is by instruction from a master, and equipment is far from being standardised. Nevertheless, the instruction given in this handbook should provide the necessary scientific background to enable newcomers to electromyography to learn the art for themselves.

J A Simpson

Preface

The purpose of this book is to provide a concise account of clinical electromyography for those working in the fields of neurology, physical medicine, and orthopaedic surgery who are likely to find the methods of practical value. It is hoped that it will be useful to undergraduate and postgraduate students interested in these subjects, and also to practising physicians and surgeons who may be concerned with the management of neuromuscular disorders.

Together with electroencephalography, electromyography has developed out of neurophysiology, but it is only in the past two decades that it has become recognised as a separate discipline widely used in clinical diagnosis. The term electromyography was originally used to refer to the methods employed to record action potentials from human muscle fibres in health and disease. In recent years, the expression has had a wider use, and is now frequently used to refer to the whole range of electrodiagnostic techniques as they are applied to peripheral nerve and muscle. It is in this sense that the expression is used in the title of this book. The field is a growing one and includes, apart from electromyography in the strict sense, the techniques of neuromuscular stimulation, which were found to be of particular value in the war years in the investigation of peripheral nerve injuries. In the past decade the study of peripheral neuropathies has been enlarged and clarified by developments in nerve conduction velocity measurement. At the same time there has been increasing interest in quantitative methods of electrodiagnosis which have contributed to the development of more objective tests.

The first six chapters contain a description of the methods and apparatus used. In this section the standard methods in general use are described, but more recent quantitative methods are also considered and an attempt has been made to indicate some of the underlying physiological principles. The remaining chapters are devoted to a review of some of the clinical conditions where electrical diagnostic methods may be of value. In these sections the purpose has been to indicate the circumstances in which electromyography may be useful, to select appropriate techniques, and to discuss the significance and limitations of the findings. The emphasis throughout has been clinical and the role of electromyography in studying the action of particular muscles in the control of posture and movement has not been discussed. The subject matter has been confined to the study of peripheral nerve and muscle, and no mention has been made of the electrical activity of the brain which belongs to the separate discipline of electroencephalography. The terminology used has been largely based on the recommendations in the Pavia Committee on Electromyography Subcommittee Report (Simpson, 1969).

The book as a whole is intended as a practical guide and not an exhaustive review, and no attempt has been made to include a complete bibliography. It is hoped, however, that sufficient references are given to provide the reader with some access to original sources. Although we have tried to draw, wherever possible, from personal experience we cannot but be conscious of our debt to others, particularly to those who have carried out the studies on which present knowledge is based.

In particular we are grateful to Professor J. A. Simpson for contributing the Foreword, for reading the manuscript, for providing Fig 10.1 and Plate 13, and many helpful suggestions. We should like to thank Dr Michael Robertson and Dr Alison Fleming for reading portions of the manuscript. The ocular electromyograms were carried out with the collaboration of Dr I. M. Strachan and Dr D. K. Whyte. The electromyographic and nerve conduction recordings were made with the technical assistance of Mrs Catherine Kinnear. The work of preparing the manuscript was carried out by Miss Joan Lindsay and Mrs Margaret Macalister, and many of the illustrations were prepared with the assistance of Mr Robert Cochrane and Mr Michael Anderson. We are glad to acknowledge the courtesy of the Medical Research Council and H.M. Stationary Office for permission to reproduce previously published material and the editors of the Proceedings of the Royal Society of Medicine for permission to reproduce Fig. 11.2. It is a pleasure to thank Mr Ian Herbert and Mr Michael Jackson and the staff of Pitman Medical Publishing Co. for their help, patience, and cooperation.

March 1969   JARL
                                                        AER

1
Electrodiagnostic Methods: Their Background and Application

Although electrodiagnostic techniques for the study of nerve and muscle have developed out of electrophysiological methods established in the course of the past hundred years it is only since the Second World War that they have achieved widespread use in clinical diagnosis. Detailed accounts already exist of the historical background (Licht, 1961; Buchthal and Rosenfalck, 1966).

Since nerve and muscle are inaccessible from the surface, their function can be studied only by the recognition of appropriate clinical signs. The application of procedures of electrical stimulation and recording depends on known physiological features of transmission and excitability and allows additional physical signs to be elicited which, in many instances, are objective and exact. At present, the procedures in use fall into two categories: (1) The artificial electrical stimulation of nerve and muscle by means of applied electric currents, and (2) the recording of the potentials that occur when nerve and muscle are active.

The electrical stimulation of nerve and muscle has given rise to two techniques. First, there is the application of stimulation techniques to determine the excitability of the tissue under study. Since muscle is normally excited through its motor nerve, and since nerve and muscle differ in their excitability, this method has been of value in deciding whether or not a muscle is properly innervated. Many different techniques have been developed to show this difference in excitability. At present, the test most commonly used is to plot the strength or intensity-duration curve using a stimulator that will produce rectangular pulses of known amplitude and duration (*see* Chapter 5). This form of test was first described in 1916 by Adrian, but the clinical application depends on the much earlier observation that denervated muscle will respond to galvanic (long duration) shocks but not to faradic (short duration) shocks. Before the advent of electronic stimulators the galvanic-faradic test, which could be performed with simple apparatus, was widely practised.

More recently, the measurement of 'accommodation', the property of excitable tissues to oppose or resist a gradually increasing stimulus, has become practicable as a clinical procedure with modern electronic apparatus (*see* Chapter 6). Here again, normal and denervated muscle can be distinguished quantitatively.

A further application of stimulation techniques has been the measurement of conduction velocity along peripheral nerves (*see* Chapter 4). This was first accomplished by Helmholtz (1850) but its clinical application was not recognised until animal experiments (Berry *et al.*, 1944; Sanders and Whitteridge, 1946) showed that conduction velocity is slowed in nerves regenerating after nerve injury. This method has since been widely applied to the study of peripheral nerve disorders.

The recording of potentials when nerve and muscle are active includes the study of evoked potentials, which are regularly recorded during nerve conduction measurements, and the study of action potentials that arise in muscle during spontaneous or voluntary activity. Although human action potentials had already been recorded many years previously, the earliest extensive study of the human electromyogram was made by Piper (1912), who recorded potentials during voluntary contraction using surface electrodes and a string galvanometer. With modern apparatus, this technique has provided much information regarding the anatomy and mode of action of different muscles in the body. In 1929, Adrian and Bronk introduced the concentric needle electrode which made it possible to study the action potentials of motor units and of single muscle fibres. Together with the development of the cathode-ray oscilloscope and electronic recording apparatus this made it possible for electromyography to develop as a clinical method (*see* Chapter 2).

These techniques form the basis of electrodiagnosis as it exists today. In recent years, many refinements have been developed, and in many instances quantitative analysis of the data obtained has become possible. Essentially, they all clarify different aspects of the functioning of the motor unit and in this way assist in understanding the disordered physiology of nerve and muscle.

THE MOTOR UNIT

The motor unit consists of an 'individual motor nerve cell and the bunch of muscle fibres it activates' (Sherrington, 1929). This complex, which consists of the nerve cell, the nerve fibre and its terminal

branches, the neuromuscular junctions, and the muscle fibres and
their constituent myofibrils, is the final pathway through which
nervous activity gives rise to voluntary movement (Fig. 1.1). The

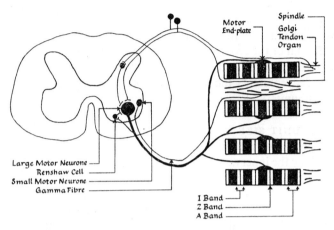

FIGURE 1.1 Diagram illustrating the innervation of the motor unit. Large
anterior horn cells is shown supplying four striated muscle fibres. Muscle spindles
lie in parallel with the muscle fibres, and afferents from the spindles act on the
large motor neurones through a single synapse. The intrafusal muscle fibres
within the spindles receive motor innervation from the small neurones in the
spinal cord through the gamma efferents. The golgi tendon organs lie in series
with the striated muscle fibres and make connection with the anterior horn cells
through a single internuncial neurone.

function of electromyography is to study the integrity of different
portions of the motor unit; at present it provides little information
regarding the central activation of the motor units although electrical
methods have been applied to the study of reflex action.

THE MOTOR UNIT POTENTIAL

When a muscle is explored with a concentric electrode and action
potentials are recorded during a voluntary contraction, the potentials
recorded are generally described as motor unit potentials. They
represent potentials derived from groups of muscle fibres that are
contracting nearly synchronously, and are situated fairly close
together and frequently activated by a single neurone. A single
electrode will record from a limited number of fibres only, and the
action potential represents the summated potentials derived from

up to about thirty fibres in the vicinity of the electrode tip (Buchthal, 1960). The motor units of the limb muscles generally contain a substantially larger number of fibres than this, and studies in which the spatial distribution of the potentials arising from a single unit has been measured with a multilead electrode indicate that the fibres of a unit are arranged in groups or subunits distributed over 5 to 10 mm of the cross section of the muscle (Buchthal *et al.*, 1959). It is likely that the action potential, or spike recorded by a single electrode, represents the summated potentials derived from one of these subunits.

MOTOR UNIT SIZE

An approximate measure of the size of motor units within a muscle is given by the innervation ratio, that is the ratio between the number of muscle fibres in a muscle and the number of motor nerves supplying it. There are many pitfalls, however, in the exact determination of motor unit size but it is clear from comparison of the results of a variety of histological and electrical techniques that the number of histological and electrical techniques that the number of fibres in a unit varies from less than twenty in the external eye muscles to more than a thousand in the muscles of the limbs.

MOTOR POINT AND END-PLATE ZONE

The motor nerve endings are not uniformly distributed throughout the muscle but are concentrated in one or more circumscribed zones known as the end-plate zones. These generally lie near the central portion of the fibres. When a muscle is excited through the skin with an electrical impulse, the stimulus is most effective when it is applied to a small localised area on the surface of the muscle. This site is known as the motor point and it corresponds to the point at which the nerve enters the muscle. Generally, the motor point lies close to the end-plate zone (Coërs and Woolf, 1959).

FAST AND SLOW UNITS

It is possible to divide motor units into fast and slow units, depending on the time the fibres of the unit take to achieve their peak tension. In many animals the muscle fibres of the fast and slow units can be distinguished by their appearance, the fibres of the slow units corresponding to the red fibres that are rich in myoglobin and the fast units to the white fibres. The red fibres are often rich in oxidative enzymes whereas white muscle may be rich in phosphorylase. This correspondence between speed of contraction and morphological character is more marked in some species than in others, and in man it is not easy to distinguish fibre types by their colour (Sissons, 1964). The speed of contraction of motor units has been shown to depend on their innervation because, if the nerves supplying fast and slow fibres are transposed, the contraction time of the slow muscle becomes rapid, and vice versa (Buller et al., 1960). At present it is not possible to distinguish between fast and slow units by electromyography in the human subject, although Tokizane has argued that the variability in spike frequency recorded from fast units during weak contractions is greater than that recorded from slow units (Tokizane and Shimazu, 1964).

RECRUITMENT AND FIRING FREQUENCY

The tension of a contracting muscle depends on the number of motor units that have been recruited and on their frequency of firing. It is probable that recruitment is the more important factor since the rate of firing of units varies between fairly narrow limits. While the frequency of nerve impulse transmission in motor nerves may range from 5 to 100 a second, it is doubtful if frequencies greater than 50 a second occur under normal circumstances. Moreover, there is evidence that each unit has a relatively restricted range of frequency, and that particular units having a particular firing frequency are recruited at different tensions. The relationship between the frequency of unit firing and the tension in a muscle is not linear but takes the form of an S-shaped curve (Bigland and Lippold, 1954).

THE MUSCLE FIBRE

The transmission of the nerve impulse and the passage of the impulse from nerve to muscle is discussed in Chapter 11. The anatomical arrangement of the muscle fibres of the motor units is that they lie in bundles but there is overlapping of units within the bundles, so that a bundle may contain fibres from more than one unit. The muscle fibres are themselves divided into many bundles of closely packed myofibrils. These are the units that undergo the process of contraction, and they are made up of thick and thin filaments which lie in parallel and can be identified under the electron microscope. The thick filaments are composed of the protein myosin and the thin filaments of actin. The thick and thin filaments are arranged so that they interdigitate, and there is evidence that during muscular contraction they slide in parallel so that the muscle shortens (Huxley and Niedergerke, 1954; Huxley and Hanson, 1954).

Cross striations have been recognised in muscle fibres for more than a hundred years and they are visible because different zones of the fibre have different refractive indices. Under the light microscope, a dark band of high refractive index known as the Z band can be identified; this divides the myofibril into segments or sarcomeres which are the functional units of the fibril. Each sarcomere contains a dark band of high refractive index known as the A band and a lighter band of low refractive index or I band. The I bands, which are each bisected by a Z band, contain thin filaments only. The A bands are the region where the interdigitating thick and thin filaments overlap.

THE MUSCLE SPINDLES AND ORGANISATION OF MOVEMENT
The central control of voluntary movement is complex and there is evidence that there are two important modes of activation of the motor units. In the first place, a rapid voluntary contraction may be initiated by direct activation of the large anterior horn cells that innervate the motor units. On the other hand, a steady sustained contraction may be initiated indirectly by activation of the small motor neurones or gamma efferents that supply the intrafusal fibres within the muscle spindles (Eldred et al., 1953). This sets up a reflex discharge in the monosynaptic pathway which activates the anterior horn cells, and contraction of the muscle is initiated.

The muscle spindles, which are sensitive to stretch, are situated in parallel with the striated muscle fibres, and are connected to the cord by a complex system of efferent and afferent fibres. They subserve both the tonic stretch reflex in response to continuous stretch and the phasic stretch reflex evoked by sudden stretch, as in the tendon jerk, and it is probable that specific parts of the spindle and specific types of nerve fibre are concerned in these different reflexes. When a muscle contracts, tension is taken off the spindle unless the spindle also shortens. Shortening of the spindle is brought about by contraction of the intrafusal fibres and in this way the gamma efferents control the sensitivity of the stretch reflex. Initiating a voluntary contraction by activating the small motor neurones and setting up a stretch reflex by causing the intrafusal fibres to shorten allows a delicate control of voluntary movement since contraction of the muscle takes the tension off the spindles and the reflex discharge ceases unless central activation continues (Boyd, 1964; Brown and Matthews, 1966). A second set of receptors lies in series with the muscle fibres. These are the Golgi tendon organs which discharge when the tension in a muscle reaches a certain level. They inhibit the large motor neurones and so may bring the stretch reflex to an end. A further arrangement exists which assists in maintaining a smooth voluntary contraction. This is a system of collateral branches of the motor neurones which connect with neurones known as Renshaw cells, which make contact with and inhibit the anterior horn cells (Renshaw, 1941). The effect of this Renshaw loop, under normal circumstances, is probably to reduce synchronous firing and prevent excessive discharge rates of motor neurones (Fig. 1.1).

METHODS OF ELECTRODIAGNOSIS

NEUROMUSCULAR STIMULATION

(a) Excitability of Nerve and Muscle
It has long been known that human muscle, where the nerve supply has been recently destroyed, can be distinguished from normal muscle by stimulation through the unbroken skin (Erb, 1883), and this distinction can be made by a variety of methods. The principle underlying these methods is that nerve and muscle differ in their excitability; hence, stimuli that will activate a normal muscle through its nerve supply are ineffective to stimulate a denervated muscle. The technique that has proven most satisfactory and is in widest use is the recording of the intensity-duration relationship of applied electrical stimuli (*see* Chapter 5). Originally shown by Adrian (1916) to be applicable to human nerve injury, modern apparatus has made it into a straightforward and reliable investigation (Ritchie, 1954). The principle of the examination is simple and fundamental, namely, that a short-duration stimulus will depolarise at a high intensity, and a long-lasting shock at a much lower or threshold strength. The relationship between the strength of a stimulus and its duration in time, for constant response of an excitable tissue, gives an accurate measure of the excitability of that tissue, and is referred to as the strength-duration or intensity-duration curve. The practical application of this method lies in the fact that denervated muscle requires a pulse of longer duration and greater intensity to effect stimulation.

The accommodation of a tissue to a stimulus of gradually increasing intensity is another property of excitable tissue which enables a distinction to be made between denervated and normal muscle, since nerve will accommodate to a far greater extent than muscle alone (*see* Chapter 6). Accommodation testing has been employed much less frequently than the intensity-duration curve but is a method of considerable theoretical promise.

(b) Nerve Conduction Measurement

Animal experiments have shown that, following denervation produced by crushing a peripheral nerve, regeneration is accompanied by slowing of conduction along the distal segment of the nerve (Sanders and Whitteridge, 1946). Likewise, in the human subject nerve injury is followed by slowing of conduction velocity. Slowing of nerve conduction may be evident less than a week after nerve injury and, generally, gradually returns to normal during the process of recovery. In severe injuries, however, where nerve suture has been carried out, some slowing of conduction may persist after clinical recovery (Hodes *et al.*, 1948). Pressure on a peripheral nerve may affect conduction velocity at this site of compression, and impairment of conduction velocity is a frequent finding in peripheral neuritis. In anterior horn cell lesions, on the other hand, there is little impairment of nerve conduction velocity since the axons of unaffected neurones continue to conduct at a normal rate. Two techniques of measurement have proved to be of value (*see also* Chapter 4).

(i) *Motor Nerve Conduction Velocity.* If the motor nerve to the hand or foot is stimulated with a short duration pulse, the potential evoked in a muscle may be displayed on a cathode-ray tube. If the stimulus is allowed to trigger the oscilloscope sweep, the latent period can be measured. If the nerve is stimulated at different points and the latencies subtracted the conduction velocity can be calculated.

(ii) *Sensory Nerve Action Potentials.* If the digital nerves at a finger are stimulated through the skin, a sensory nerve action potential can be recorded at the wrist or elbow. It is of low amplitude, 20 μV or smaller, and less easy to record than an evoked muscle potential, but abnormalities in amplitude or latency provide a very delicate sign of a peripheral nerve lesion (Gilliatt and Sears, 1958). A modified technique is to stimulate a nerve peripherally and record the mixed sensory and antidromic motor nerve potential proximally.

Of great value in the diagnosis of peripheral nerve injuries and of many varieties of peripheral neuropathy, nerve conduction velocity studies have been particularly helpful in the recognition of lesions due to local pressure on peripheral nerves.

ELECTROMYOGRAPHY

Electromyography is a method of studying the activity of a muscle by recording action potentials from the contracting fibres (see Chapter 2). This can be done through surface electrodes applied to the overlying skin, but for diagnostic purposes it is useful to employ concentric needle electrodes which are inserted through the skin into the muscle (Adrian and Bronk, 1929). These consist of a hollow needle surrounding an insulated wire core which is bared at the tip. Such an electrode will record potentials from muscle fibres in its vicinity which, after amplification, are displayed on a cathode-ray tube and frequently reproduced through a loudspeaker. Electromyography has been of value in the analysis of the actions of different muscles in the maintenance of posture (Joseph, 1960; Basmajian, 1968) and in the study of the physiology of motor unit activity (Bigland and Lippold, 1954). The clinical applications have been principally in the diagnosis and prognostic assessment of peripheral nerve lesions, in the differentiation and detailed study of peripheral neuropathies and diseases affecting voluntary muscle, and in the recognition of anterior horn cell disease.

CLINICAL APPLICATIONS

DENERVATION

Loss of continuity between the nerve fibre and a skeletal muscle can be recognised by means of the strength-duration curve, by nerve conduction measurement, and by electromyography. These three methods are complementary, since they each provide information of a specific character, but which will be most valuable depends on the particular clinical situation.

Following a nerve injury, the strength-duration curve becomes abnormal within a few days, which may constitute the earliest objective sign of denervation. In recovering lesions, the strength duration curve frequently gives advance information of reinnervation before any voluntary contraction of the muscle can be seen. On the other hand, although it is of value in early diagnosis and in prognosis, this method gives little information regarding the underlying pathology.

Nerve conduction measurement is of relatively limited value in the recognition of partial denervation since it may be normal, the presence or absence of conduction delay depending on the nature of the pathology affecting the nerve. In complete denervation, on the other hand, the test may be helpful since, after division of a peripheral nerve, all conduction in the distal segment may cease before the end of the first week. Failure to detect an evoked potential in a muscle after stimulation of its motor nerve may thus be an early sign of denervation. This sign is particularly useful when applied to the facial nerve (*see* Chapter 8).

Electromyography may also provide evidence of denervation. If a muscle is explored with a concentric electrode the sign that it may be denervated is the presence of small potentials which occur spontaneously in relaxed muscle and which are known as fibrillation potentials. These potentials may not occur until as late as three weeks after nerve injury. Electromyography does not, therefore, provide such early evidence of denervation as is provided by other methods, but it provides more information regarding the extent and nature of the pathology. Thus, sampling different parts of the muscle with a concentric electrode may indicate the extent of the denervation and how much of the muscle is functioning normally. If some voluntary activity remains, the character of the motor unit potentials may indicate the nature of the underlying pathology. Its value in prognosis is of the same order as the strength-duration curve, and during reinnervation after complete nerve section it may be possible to detect voluntary units by electromyography before voluntary movement is visible (*see* Chapter 7).

DISORDERS OF NERVE CELL AND AXON

Electromyography and nerve conduction velocity measurement used together are of particular value in analysing the nature of peripheral nerve disease. Fibrillation potentials may be seen both in anterior horn cell disease and in peripheral neuropathies but the type of voluntary motor unit potentials recorded may differ in the two conditions. Although in both conditions there is reduced motor unit activity and sometimes an excess of polyphasic potentials, in anterior horn cell disease many of the potentials are of abnormally large amplitude and duration and there is a tendency for them to fire synchronously. Nerve conduction velocity is slowed down when the integrity of the myelin sheaths of the nerves is impaired. It is, therefore, predominantly affected in those peripheral neuropathies where the primary damage is to the myelin sheath. Where axonal damage follows changes in the neurone, as in certain of the toxic neuropathies, conduction velocity may be slowed but to a lesser degree. Where anterior horn cells are selectively destroyed, as in poliomyelitis or motor nuerone disease, conduction velocity may remain normal so long as the axons of a few unaffected neurones remain intact; where the motor axons of a mixed trunk have all been lost it may still be possible to record conduction in the sensory axons. In these circumstances, careful analysis of electromyographic and conduction measurement results may contribute significantly to the diagnosis (see Chapter 9).

NEUROMUSCULAR BLOCK

While myasthenia gravis is the most important condition in which neuromuscular block is a feature, the neuromuscular junction may also be affected in polymyositis and the myasthenic syndrome associated with bronchial carcinoma and a degree of neuromuscular block may occur in cases of peripheral neuropathy. The widespread use of muscle relaxants in anaesthesia has aroused interest in the pharmacology of neuromuscular transmission. In all these conditions, but primarily in myasthenia gravis, the study of the effect of repetitive nerve stimulation on the size of evoked muscle potentials has contributed usefully to understanding of the disorder and in some measure also to practical diagnosis (see Chapter 11).

MUSCLE DISEASE

The finding of an abnormal strength-duration curve or delayed nerve conduction may indicate the presence of denervation or of a peripheral nerve lesion and so make the diagnosis of a myopathy in a patient less likely. These tests, however, do not provide positive evidence of a myopathy. In this respect, electromyography is of particular value since the motor unit pattern of myopathic muscle is distinctive. This motor unit pattern is common both to the genetically determined muscular dystrophies and to the acquired forms of myopathy such as polymyositis, thyrotoxic, and drug induced myopathy. In certain cases of polymyositis, however, the presence of profuse spontaneous electrical activity in relaxed muscle may serve to distinguish the condition from muscular dystrophy. In the myotonias, the occurrence of high-frequency discharges during relaxation from a voluntary contraction or following mechanical stimulation by the electrode provides a valuable confirmatory sign in doubtful cases.

In recent years, the development of quantitative techniques of electromyography has contributed significantly to the study of muscle disease. Of particular interest has been the application of electromyography to the detection of clinically unaffected carriers of muscular dystrophy, and the methods that have been developed in this connection include refractory period measurement, the measurement of mean action potential duration, and the computer analysis of spike counts (*see* Chapters 3 and 10).

SPASTIC STATES

Although action potentials may be more readily evoked from spastic muscle by passive movement than from healthy muscle, in general, electromyography has given little information regarding lesions affecting the upper motor neurone. One method, which has been widely studied, is the determination of excitability of the H reflex (*see* Chapter 4). The H reflex is the electrical counterpart of the ankle jerk, and the conditions under which it can be evoked give an indication of the excitability of that part of the motor neurone pool concerned in the phasic stretch reflex. It has been found that, if the H reflex is evoked repetitively with paired stimuli, the excitability of the reflex shows a characteristic recovery cycle during the 1,000 msec after the reflex is obtained. Between 10 and 100 msec after a first reflex, a second reflex cannot be obtained, and thereafter it takes a significant period to revert to its previous size. This recovery cycle is altered in the presence of clinical spasticity and in Parkinson's disease. This method is time-consuming and great care and attention to technical detail is necessary to obtain reproducible results. It has not, as yet, achieved routine use as a diagnostic method but it provides a possible approach to the study of central nervous system disorders.

ELECTROMYOGRAPHY IN PAEDIATRICS

An adequate electromyographic examination depends on the full co-operation of the patient, who must be able to contract and relax his muscles in a controlled manner at the request of the examiner. In very young children this degree of co-operation is not always obtained when the examination is one that includes needle puncture.

For this reason, the most reliable information is obtained in studying conditions where strength-duration curves or nerve conduction velocity measurement are the appropriate tests. Nerve conduction measurement is well tolerated in children and is of great value in identifying the acute case of polyneuritis and in recognising system disorders where the peripheral nerves may be affected, such as peroneal muscular atrophy, hypertrophic polyneuritis, and meta-chromatic leucodystrophy (*see* Chapter 8). In suspected cases of infantile spinal muscular atrophy (Werdnig-Hoffman's disease), electromyography may be of value as fibrillations can sometimes be identified even if it is not possible to study the motor unit pattern. Generally speaking, however, the electromyographic study of the myopathies of early infancy is a matter of some difficulty and, frequently, uninformative. In later childhood, electromyography is of value in the recognition of the muscular dystrophies but requires patience and care, as a child will not readily tolerate the sampling, with a needle electrode, of several sites in a group of muscles.

2
Electromyography

The study of the electrical activity of contracting muscle provides information concerning the structure and functioning of the motor units. This may make it possible to localise the site of pathology affecting either muscle or its innervation and, in addition, may frequently provide evidence regarding the nature of the pathological process.

The nerve fibres that supply muscle are each the extension of a neurone within the grey matter of the brain or spinal cord, and they each give off terminal branches which supply a large number of muscle fibres. The nerve cell and the muscle fibres it supplies is defined as the motor unit. Whenever a muscle fibre contracts, the surface membrane undergoes depolarisation so that an action potential can be recorded from the fibre. When the fibres of a motor unit are activated, they contract nearly, but not quite, synchronously, and their action potentials summate so that a relatively large complex potential, known as the motor unit action potential, can be recorded.

In disease in which the structure and function of the motor unit is affected, the motor unit action potentials may have an abnormal configuration and the pattern of motor unit activity during voluntary contraction may be altered. In health, muscle fibres contract only when they are activated by neurones and, hence, under normal conditions it is only motor unit action potentials that are seen. In neuromuscular disease, however, single muscle fibres may contract apparently spontaneously, and this may be recognised by the appearance of action potentials derived from single muscle fibres or from very small groups of fibres. Electromyography is the technique by which the action potentials of contracting muscle fibres and motor units are recorded and displayed.

APPARATUS AND TECHNIQUE
The action potential of a single muscle fibre can be recorded in isolation if a microelectrode is used to impale the muscle fibre

14

(*see* Chapter 3) As the electrode enters the fibre it becomes negative to the outside of the fibre by about 90 mV. The recording apparatus records this potential difference across the cell membrane as the resting membrane potential. When the muscle is activated, the potential difference across the cell membrane is reversed, so that for a short space of time the outside of the membrane becomes negative and the inside positive, and the recording system registers the changes in potential as the action potential, which recorded in this way, may be greater than 100 mV. Microelectrodes used for recording from single cells are usually made from glass tubing drawn to a fine point of the order of 0·50 μ in diameter and filled with KCl solution. This technique has proved valuable in the study of experimental animals but cannot readily be applied to human muscle and is not at present suitable for routine clinical use.

In clinical practice, muscle action potentials are usually recorded by extracellular electrodes placed in close proximity to the muscle fibres. When this is done, the potentials are very much smaller than those recorded by intracellular electrodes and range from about 15 μV to about 10 mV. Amplification is therefore necessary before the potentials can be displayed on a cathode-ray oscilloscope. For the detailed study of motor unit activity it is necessary to use needle electrodes which can be inserted into the substance of the muscle to lie between the fibres. Electrical activity can also be recorded from electrodes placed on the skin overlying the muscle but if this is done the potentials recorded are the summated potentials derived from many motor units. Surface electrodes, however, are of value when one wishes to record the amount of electrical activity associated with a muscular contraction and when it is not necessary to study the character of individual motor unit potentials.

Under normal circumstances, if extracellular electrodes are used, the action potentials of single fibres are not seen since, during voluntary contraction, fibres are activated in groups so that the potentials recorded are motor unit action potentials. Single fibre potentials may, however, be recorded in certain pathological conditions where muscle fibres contract spontaneously and give rise to isolated discharges. Under normal circumstances single motor unit action potentials can be recorded satisfactorily only during weak contractions since, during a powerful contraction, so many are activated that many of the potentials occur synchronously and give rise to an interference pattern on the oscilloscope screen. If single unit potentials are to be recorded during a strong contraction it is necessary to employ fine-wire electrodes with a particularly small tip which will record only from the unit in which it is placed.

RECORDING ELECTRODES
The varieties of electrode commonly used in clinical electromyography are described below.

(a) *Surface Electrodes*
These are generally small plates made of silver or stainless steel which may be placed in pairs over a muscle so that the potential difference between them may be recorded. One electrode can be at earth potential, but it is frequently more satisfactory to connect each electrode to one side of a balanced amplifier, a third lead connecting the patient to ground.

(b) *Concentric Needle Electrodes*
These are the electrodes at present most widely employed in clinical electromyography. They consist of a pointed cannula, similar to a hypodermic needle, in the core of which is cemented an insulated

a

b

FIGURE 2.1 Concentric electrodes (a) unipolar, (b) bipolar.

wire made of stainless steel or platinum, which is bare at the tip (Fig. 2.1). The potential difference between the bare tip of the central wire and the outer cannula is recorded, and the cannula is generally grounded. Concentric electrodes can be readily constructed in the laboratory (Silver, 1958), but are manufactured in a variety of sizes; for many purposes a needle of 24 s.w.g. is suitable but for insertion into the muscles of the face or the extra-ocular muscles a thickness of 30 s.w.g. or less is appropriate.

(c) Bipolar Needle Electrodes
These consist of a cannula containing two insulated wires with bare tips (Fig. 2.1). With this electrode the potential difference between the two bare wires can be recorded, and a satisfactory arrangement is to connect the two central wires to the two sides of a balanced amplifier, while the outer cannula is earthed. Bipolar electrodes may also usefully be employed as stimulating electrodes.

(d) Monopolar Needle Electrodes
These are solid electrodes coated with insulating varnish and bared at the tip. The voltage changes are recorded between this electrode and a separate reference electrode which may be a metal plate on the surface of the skin or a second needle in the subcutaneous tissue. Needles of this kind, which can be inserted directly through the skin, are best made from good quality stainless-steel wire with the tip ground to a fine point. They can also be quite readily adapted from steel sewing needles. An alternative arrangement is to use fine insulated stainless-steel wire of about 40 s.w.g. which may be inserted through the core of a hypodermic needle. The tip of such an electrode can be made so fine that it will record from a very small area only, and will, therefore, allow single unit potentials to be recorded even during a powerful voluntary contraction.

(e) Mutilead Electrodes
These are electrodes that contain at least three insulated wires within a common steel cannula. In the usual form, the tips of the wires appear at intervals along the side of the cannula. One form of multilead electrode has been extensively employed to study the extent of the territory occupied by the fibres of a single motor unit (Buchthal *et al.*, 1959). Another variety of multi-electrode has been developed to stimulate and record from single muscle fibres (Ekstedt, 1964).

(f) Intracellular Electrodes
If an electrode is to penetrate a single cell and register the potential changes across the membrane, it must have an exceedingly fine tip with a diameter of the order of 0·50 μ (Fig. 2.2).

3

Electrodes of this kind are usually drawn from fine Pyrex glass tubing and are filled with 3 Molar potassium chloride solution. They have a high resistance, generally in excess of 5 MΩ and must, therefore, be connected to recording equipment with a particularly high input impedance. They are easily broken and must be

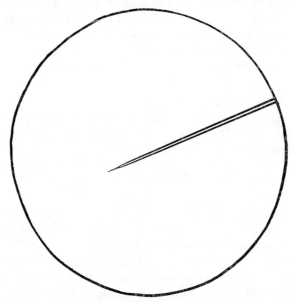

FIGURE 2.2 Glass microelectrode viewed through low power microscope (X100). The tip of the electrode has a diameter of about 0·5 μ and can only be resolved with the electron microscope. The size of the electrode tip is normally estimated by measuring the resistance of the electrode.

inserted by a micromanipulator, either into the exposed surface of a muscle, or through the skin, using an outer cannula to penetrate the tissue (Beranek, 1964). Glass microelectrodes will not keep more than a few days and, therefore, have to be made for each occasion they are used (Kennard, 1958).

THE AMPLIFICATION AND DISPLAY OF THE
ELECTROMYOGRAM

The electric changes recorded by the electrodes represent voltages ranging from a few microvolts to more than 10 mV, and these must therefore be amplified before they can be displayed for analysis.

After amplification they are generally displayed on the screen of a cathode-ray oscilloscope where they may be observed and photographed. In clinical practice, the ear can identify certain features of the electromyogram more readily than the eye, so it is of value to have a simultaneous auditory record of the potential changes through a loudspeaker. Storage of the changes on magnetic tape enables samples of the electromyogram to be played again through the loudpseaker or displayed repeatedly on the oscilloscope. A polaroid camera is useful for photographing single oscilloscope sweeps, as may be done when measuring action potential duration or studying evoked potentials. For continuous records of the electromyogram it is useful to have a camera that will photograph a stationary spot on moving film.

The characteristics of the amplifying system are important if the voltage changes arising from muscle are to be accurately recorded. While surface electrodes can be applied after careful preparation of the skin so that there is little resistance between the electrode and the patient, needle and wire electrodes may have a relatively high resistance. If the muscle is regarded as a source of voltage, the greater part of the internal resistance of this voltage source is derived from the resistance of the electrodes. This internal resistance leads to a loss of voltage between the source and the recording apparatus, which is also dependent on the input resistance of the amplifier. In this context we are concerned with potentials that are changing continuously, so that the expression impedance, which refers to alternating current, is more appropriate than resistance. If R is the input impedance and r is the source impedance (equivalent to the electrode impedance), the proportion of the voltage transferred from the source to the recording apparatus is $R/(r + R)$. Thus, if the input impedance is more than twenty times the source impedance the voltage loss will be negligible. Since both the source and input impedance depend on capacitance as well as resistance, they are both frequency dependent, the impedance in each case decreasing with higher frequencies.

With surface electrodes carefully applied, the resistance between the electrodes and the skin should not be greater than $10,000 \ \Omega$ and the input impedance of the recorder need not be greater than $1 \ M\Omega$ to prevent loss of signal strength, even if there are large fluctuations in interelectrode resistance. On the other hand, fine wire electrodes, particularly if the tips are ground to a fine point, may have a resistance of as much as 1MΩ or greater (Buchthal *et al.*, 1954), so that for some purposes it may be necessary to use an amplifier with an input impedance of 20 to 100 MΩ. With concentric electrodes, although the resistance is higher than that of surface electrodes, it is considerably less than that of fine unipolar electrodes, so that for most purposes in clinical practice an input impedance of 5 to 20 MΩ is adequate. Excessively long, shielded cables between the electrode and the amplifier effectively increase the input capacitance and so lower the input impedance, especially at high frequencies (Rogoff and Reiner, 1961).

The higher the resistance of the recording electrode the more likely it is to pick up interference from external electrical sources such as the mains, and for this reason it is most satisfactory to record the electromyogram with a balanced amplifier. The principle of this is that the electrode terminals are connected into opposite halves of the amplifier so that when one input terminal goes positive the other goes negative, whenever there is a potential difference between the electrodes. Outside interference, however, will affect both sides of the amplifier in the same way and this 'in phase' signal is not amplified. The ability of a balanced amplifier to discriminate between 'in phase' and 'out of phase' signals is termed its rejection ratio. While suitable recording equipment assists greatly in reducing interference, it is important also to keep the recording leads as short as possible, to make certain that all external connections are sound, that the patient is earthed, and that all earth connections terminate in a single site which has a low resistance connection to ground. It is seldom necessary to introduce elaborate screening arrangements but, occasionally, if the laboratory is close to some powerful external source of interference such as diathermy, it may be necessary to enclose the room in an earthed wire screen or, alternatively, to employ a Faraday cage to screen the patient.

If it is intended to measure the amplitude and duration of the action potentials it is important to display them as far as possible without distortion, and this means that the amplifier must have an adequate response. While an upper frequency response of about 50,000 c/s is necessary to record rapid transients without distortion, the majority of the potentials that appear on the electromyogram can be adequately reproduced with recording apparatus that responds to frequencies of 2 to 10,000 c/s (Buchthal, *et al.*, 1954). Although a frequency response of this order is necessary to enable potentials to be measured without distortion, in practice it is possible to recognise the more important characteristics of the electromyogram with a more restricted frequency response.

An inherent limitation of all amplification systems is that they are subject to noise. This is so described because it may be heard on the loudspeaker as a continuous background hiss, which at high amplification of very small signals may obscure the signal. It is due to random fluctuations in the system and consists of source noise, which depends on the magnitude of the source resistance and its temperature and is irreducible so long as these factors are constant, and amplifier noise which can be reduced to some extent by appropriate design of the equipment. Both forms of noise are evenly distributed over a wide frequency band extending to many megacycles a second, so the amount of noise can be markedly reduced by restricting the band width. A good quality amplifier may give rise to less than 5 μV of noise at 10,000 c/s, which allows the smaller potentials seen in electromyography to be adequately displayed.

In the study of evoked nerve action potentials, a low noise level is particularly important as these potentials may be less than 5 μV in amplitude. Measures that may make it possible to record these very small potentials include reducing the frequency response to as low as 1,000 c/s (Plate 1), using an input transformer between the preparation and the recording equipment to increase the signal-to-noise ratio (Buchthal and Rosenfalck, 1965), and photographing repetitive superimposed traces so that a regularly recurring signal appears enhanced, whereas the random noise is unchanged. A further refinement is to use a computer that adds and enhances a repetitively recurring signal but has no effect on the random fluctuations of background noise.

The amplification of signals from intracellular microelectrodes imposes particular problems. A glass microelectrode may have a resistance of from 3 to 100 Mμ, and this means that the amplifier should have an input impedance of the order of 10^{10} MΩ which is usually achieved by having a cathode-follower input. In addition to a high resistance, the microelectrode has a high capacitance, and the combination of a high resistance and a high capacitance in the input circuit means that the system has a long time constant which severely limits the upper frequency response. Measures that may compensate for this are to shorten the input lead by separating the input valve and its circuit from the main amplifier to bring it close to the preparation, connecting the screening of the input lead to the cathode of the input valve, and compensating for the input capacitance by incorporating a positive feedback arrangement in the amplifier. A suitable d.c. amplifier for microelectrode work will incorporate these features and, in addition, the grid current passed in the input circuit will be very small, preferably less than 10^{-12} A.

TECHNIQUE

In any electromyographic examination, unless a low temperature is required to bring out a particular abnormality such as myotonia, it is important that the limbs to be examined should be warm. If surface electrodes are used, the skin should be prepared by washing with spirit or ether and by applying electrode jelly, although these precautions are less important when amplifiers of high input impedance are used. With concentric electrodes the skin should be cleaned and sterilised with antiseptic solution. If the same concentric electrode is used on more than a single patient, particular care in sterilisation is necessary to avoid the risk of transmitting hepatitis virus. An acceptable standard is to wash each electrode thoroughly after use with water and detergent and then carry out heat sterilisation by autoclaving. An alternative to autoclaving which is less likely to cause breakdown of electrode insulation, is gas sterilisation in ethylene oxide.

The electrode is inserted into the muscle through the skin with the limb relaxed, and during insertion the presence or absence of excessive insertion activity is recorded. A search is then made in different parts of the relaxed muscle for spontaneous electrical activity. After this, the patient contracts the muscle voluntarily and the motor unit potentials during different grades of voluntary contraction are observed with the electrode at different sites within the muscle.

THE POTENTIALS RECORDED ON ELECTROMYOGRAPHY

SPONTANEOUS ACTIVITY

When a healthy muscle is relaxed, the muscle fibres are not contracting and an intramuscular electrode will record no electrical activity. Motor unit activity when it is recorded is generally a sign of incomplete relaxation, but small action potentials representing single fibres or small groups of fibres are occasionally seen in healthy subjects during relaxation when the recording electrode is placed within or close to the end-plate zone of the muscle.

In neuromuscular disease, spontaneous activity may be of clinical value. An important variety is known as fibrillation, and while this may occur sparsely in healthy muscle and is a feature of a variety of neuromuscular disorders, it is particularly characteristic of denervated muscle. Fibrillation cannot be seen as visible contraction through the skin, although it may be visible in an exposed muscle and can occasionally be recognised in the tongue. Fibrillation potentials, however, can be readily recorded with concentric electrodes, and their identification is of considerable importance in diagnosis. The important varieties of spontaneous activity seen in voluntary muscle and which can be identified by their electrical accompaniments are as follows.

(a) *Insertion Activity*

When a needle electrode is inserted into a muscle it evokes a discharge of action potentials which lasts only a brief period longer than the electrode movement. These action potentials are of short duration and small amplitude when compared with motor unit action potentials, and they are probably due to mechanical excitation of the muscle fibres by electrode movement. Although they are generally seen in normal muscle, they are particularly easily induced and tend to be prolonged in denervated muscle (Plate 2) and in muscle affected by certain muscular disorders, in particular polymyositis. Insertion activity when it occurs in neuromuscular disease may include abnormal potentials, such as positive sharp waves, which are not seen in healthy muscle (Weddell et al., 1944; Kugelberg and Petersén, 1949; Jasper and Ballem, 1949).

(b) *End-plate Noise*

This includes two types of potential that may be recorded from the end-plate zone of muscle. The first is a brief high-frequency potential of up to 2 msec duration and 100 μV amplitude which occurs as a monophasic negative discharge. These potentials are considered to represent miniature end-plate potentials recorded extracellularly. Miniature end-plate potentials are small potentials that can be recorded by an intracellular electrode inserted at the region of the end-plate. They occur continuously in random manner and are independent of the nerve impulse. In addition, diphasic potentials may be recorded from the end-plate zone which are of longer duration reaching 2 to 3 msec and with an amplitude of up to 200 μV. The nature of these potentials is uncertain. It is possible they arise from small bundles of intramuscular nerve fibres; alternatively, they may represent groups of nearly synchronous miniature end-plate potentials (Jones *et al.*, 1955; Buchthal and Rosenfalck, 1966).

(c) *Fibrillation Potentials* (Plate 2)
These are small potentials which most commonly have a duration lasting from 0·5 to 2 msec and an amplitude of 30 to 150 μV. They may be recorded from any part of a muscle but, when recorded from the end-plate zone where they may be diphasic with an initial negative deflection, they may be difficult to distinguish from end-plate noise. Elsewhere in the muscle they may have an initial positive phase, which is of value in identifying the potentials as fibrillation (Buchthal and Rosenfalck, 1966). They generally occur at a rate of 2 to 10 a second and may be diphasic or triphasic. They are probably derived from single spontaneously contracting muscle fibres, but some are of relatively large size, reaching an amplitude of 1 mV or more, and it is possible that these larger potentials represent the synchronous contraction of small groups of fibres.

Although fibrillation potentials may be observed very occasionally in healthy muscle and may also occur in certain forms of myopathy, they are particularly characteristic of denervated muscle. In lower motor neurone lesions they are a valuable sign that the continuity between the motor axon and the muscle fibre has been interrupted, but they may not appear until as long as three weeks after this has taken place. The underlying mechanism of fibrillation is not understood. It has long been known that denervated muscle is abnormally sensitive to acetyl choline (Brown, 1937) and one possible explanation is that spontaneous activity arises through the activity of small quantities of circulating acetyl choline (Denny-Brown and Pennybacker, 1938). This is supported by the observation that after denervation the whole of the muscle fibre membrane, and not merely the end-plate zone, becomes sensitive to acetyl choline (Axelsson and Thesleff, 1959). On the other hand, there is evidence that although fibrillation potentials may be recorded anywhere in a muscle they always arise in the end-plate zone and they continue to occur after the administration of curare (Thesleff, 1963; Belmar and Eyzaguirre, 1966). The physical properties of the muscle fibre membrane are altered after denervation (Nicholls, 1956), and in mammalian muscle the resting membrane potential is lowered (Lüllmann and Pracht, 1957; Lenman, 1965). In favour of the possibility that fibrillation is due to a circulating substance, not necessarily acetyl choline, is the fact that it cannot be recorded in isolated muscle (Thesleff, 1963) and it is abolished after occlusion of the blood supply to a limb (Hnik and Skorpil, 1962).

That acetyl choline sensitivity is not the main cause of fibrillation is supported by the fact that neostigmine is relatively ineffective in augmenting fibrillation. A more effective procedure is to apply a direct depolarising current to the muscle (Landau, 1951), although there are technical problems in recording small voltages in the presence of a strong external current. An important practical consideration in searching for fibrillation is that the muscle must be warm, since fibrillations disappear with moderate lowering of the temperature.

(d) *Positive Sharp Waves* (Fig. 2.3)
These potentials are of longer duration than fibrillation potentials but are of comparable voltage. They consist of an initial positive spike followed by a slow change of potential in the negative direction which may lead to a prolonged negative phase, so that the total duration may be greater than 10 msec. Because of their characteristic shape they are sometimes known as positive 'saw-tooth' potentials. These sharp waves occur repetitively and are characteristically evoked by electrode movement, forming an important feature of pathological insertion activity. They also occur, apparently, spontaneously, and frequently accompany fibrillation potentials. Their origin is not known but they probably represent the discharge of single muscle fibres and may be due to the needle electrode recording near a damaged part of a muscle fibre. They do not occur in healthy muscle and are seen most frequently in denervated muscle. In addition, they occur in polymyositis and in association with myotonia.

(e) *Fasciculation*
Fasciculations are spontaneous contractions of groups of muscle fibres or of motor units large enough to produce visible contraction of the muscle without evoking movement at the joint. They may

occur in healthy subjects and in conditions affecting the lower motor neurone such as irritation of nerve roots. Their most serious significance is when they occur in degenerative disease affecting the anterior horn cells, as for example motor neurone disease, or in syringomyelia and the acute pre-paralytic phase of poliomyelitis. It is of obvious importance to distinguish the fasciculations due to

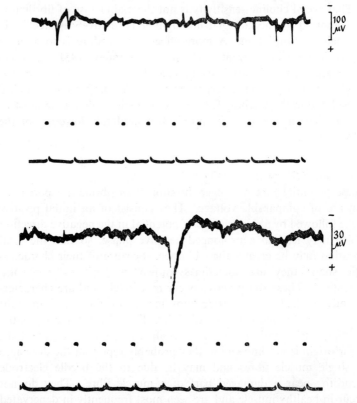

FIGURE 2.3 Positive sharp waves in partially denervated muscle. Time scale 10 msec.

anterior horn cell involvement from the so-called benign fasciculations, but this is a matter of considerable difficulty as there is nothing distinctive in appearance in the fasciculation potential. The rate of firing is a possibly significant feature and it has been suggested that the fasciculations of motor neurone disease appear at a slower rate, namely, about every three to four seconds, compared with a rate of nearly one a second with the so-called benign fasciculations (Trojaborg and Buchthal, 1965).

(*f*) *The Myotonic Response* (Plates 4 and 5)

In the myotonias a high-frequency discharge of action potentials may be evoked by electrode movement, or may follow percussion of a muscle, or may occur during relaxation from a voluntary contraction. The frequency of the discharge is variable, ranging about 10 a second to 150 a second. They are characterised by a gradual increase in frequency, after which the potentials decrease both in amplitude and rate of firing. It is this change in the frequency of the discharge that gives rise to an unmistakable sound when played through a loudspeaker, which has been likened to a dive-bomber pulling out of a dive. The individual potentials comprising the myotonic discharge show considerable variation in characteristics. Some are brief and of low amplitude and resemble fibrillation potentials, others are indistinguishable from motor unit action potentials, and potentials similar in appearance to the positive sharp waves seen in denervated muscle are frequently observed.

The recognition and identification of spontaneous potentials is of considerable value in diagnosis but calls for careful and critical technique, particularly as regards the recognition of fibrillation. The use of the loudspeaker is of particular value as fibrillation gives rise to a characteristic crackling sound. The sound of a myotonic discharge is not easily mistaken and the ear is a particularly valuable aid, especially when it comes to recognising the frequency of a discharge. One source of difficulty is that in certain muscles, particularly those of the face, such as the frontalis muscle, the motor units are of relatively small size and give rise to short duration potentials so that minimal voluntary activity can readily be confused with fibrillation. A second difficulty is that end-plate noise may be mistaken for fibrillation unless care is taken to explore the muscle widely and identify potentials outside the end-plate area. A further difficulty arises from the fact that potentials having all the characteristics of fibrillation potentials are not confined to denervated muscle. They may, for example, be seen in healthy muscle, although never profusely. Isolated fibrillation potentials not encountered in other areas of the muscle must therefore be evaluated with caution. In muscular dystrophy, fibrillation is occasionally observed, and it may be widespread and profuse in polymyositis (Walton and Adams, 1958).

(a) *The Motor Unit Action Potential*
Motor unit action potentials are the principal electrical event recorded from muscle during voluntary contraction. They consist of the summated action potentials derived from groups of muscle fibres that are contracting nearly but not quite synchronously. They may be monophasic, diphasic, or triphasic, and are occasionally polyphasic with five or more phases. The duration generally ranges from 2 to 10 msec and the amplitude from 100 μV to 2 mV The range of values obtained depends to a considerable extent on the technique and circumstances of recording. Thus, different values for amplitude and duration are obtained with concentric needle electrodes, bipolar electrodes, and unipolar electrodes. With electrodes of the same type, the size of the recording surface will affect the characteristics of the action potential, and even with electrodes of the same batch different values may be obtained with different electrodes (Buchthal *et al.*, 1954). Faithful reproduction of action potentials depends also on adequate amplifier design, and particularly important to the source impedance of the electrode and an adequate frequency response in the amplifying system. In the healthy subject, there is considerable variation between the size of the action potentials in different muscles studied (Plate 3). This probably depends on the number of fibres comprised in the motor units in particular muscles. Thus, in the external ocular muscles the motor units contain only a few muscle fibres, and the mean action potential duration is less than 2·0 msec (Björk and Kugelberg, 1953). The facial muscles contain somewhat larger units and the mean action potential duration is slightly longer, but it is considerably shorter than in the limb muscles where the motor units may contain in excess of 500 muscle fibres (Feinstein *et al.*, 1955). There is also some variation with age for, on average, mean action potential duration tends to be more prolonged the older the subject (Sacco *et al.*, 1962).

The shape and dimensions of motor unit action potentials are considerably modified by disease. In peripheral neuropathies, partial denervation frequently occurs and is followed by regeneration.

Regenerating fibres conduct their impulses more slowly than healthy axons. In addition to this, in many cases of peripheral neuropathy there is widespread slowing of nerve conduction velocity. One effect of this is that the time intervals, which already exist between the moment of activation of individual fibres in the motor units, are lengthened so that the motor unit action potential becomes prolonged and may be relatively polyphasic (Plate 6). If analysis of the action potential dimensions in peripheral neuropathy is carried out, it is generally found that the mean action potential duration is prolonged but the amplitude is normal or reduced (Buchthal and Pinelli, 1953). In addition, there is an abnormal number of polyphasic potentials. The situation is different in disease affecting the anterior horn cells in the spinal cord. Here, a proportion of the nerve cells with their associated fibres may be intact whereas others have undergone degeneration. When this happens the axons of surviving neurones send out branches to innervate muscle fibres that have lost their nerve supply. In this way the total number of motor units in the muscle is reduced but those that remain are enlarged (Wohlfart, 1958; Erminio et al., 1959; Coërs and Woolf, 1959). These large motor units may have a duration exceeding 12 msec and an amplitude of up to 10 mV (Plate 7A). Where disease affects the muscle fibres, as distinct from their nerve supply, there is no loss of motor units until the disease is far advanced. However, many of the muscle fibres that compose the motor units undergo degeneration, so that the units contain a reduced number of muscle fibres. This has the effect of, on average, reducing the mean duration of the action potentials. The amplitude of the action potentials is also slightly reduced (Buchthal and Pinelli, 1952; Pinelli and Buchthal, 1953). Because many of the fibres in the motor units have been lost, the motor unit potentials may be polyphasic and, in severe cases, this gives rise to an unmistakable crackling noise on the loudspeaker (Plate 7B).

(b) The Pattern of Voluntary Contraction

When a healthy muscle is completely relaxed no electrical activity is evident apart from the background noise of the amplifying system. During a weak voluntary contraction motor unit action potentials can be distinguished; they are clearly separated from one another so that their duration, amplitude, and shape can be distinguished. As the force of the contraction increases, more motor units are recruited so that during a strong voluntary contraction so many motor unit potentials become superimposed one upon the other that it is impossible to determine their individual characteristics. This situation is known as an interference pattern (Plates 8A and B).

When the nerve supply of a muscle is affected for any reason, it is no longer possible to recruit the maximum number of motor units during voluntary contraction, and the effect of this on the electromyogram is that the interference pattern is reduced or, in severe cases, may be lost altogether. Thus, in a severe case of neuropathic muscular weakness it is possible to identify the action potentials of individual units even during maximal contractions. This becomes particularly striking in disease affecting the anterior horn cells, when large motor units of up to 10 mV in amplitude may stand out against a background of relative electrical silence.

In myopathic disorders, on the other hand, the recruitment of motor units is unaffected although the motor units themselves are abnormal. Thus, in muscular dystrophy, during weak voluntary contraction the individual motor unit potentials can be recognised as being, in many cases, highly polyphasic. During a maximal voluntary contraction there is a full interference pattern, but, since this interference pattern is made up of motor units that are themselves polyphasic, it differs from the interference pattern of normal muscle in that the frequency distribution of electrical activity is altered in the direction of higher frequencies. This is most readily recognised by the ear when recording through a loudspeaker.

3
Quantitative Methods in Electromyography

Electromyography, as it is generally carried out relies principally on visual inspection of the potential changes displayed on the oscilloscope, and auditory interpretation of the signals when played through a loudspeaker. These may be supplemented by a permanent photographic record of the potentials. The simple data they provide is useful in a variety of neuromuscular disorders and, often, are adequate to establish or confirm a diagnosis. The method, however, remains subjective, and a great deal depends on the experience of the operator. The most generally useful advance for obtaining objective results that can be presented in a quantitative and reproducible manner has been the development of techniques for measuring nerve conduction velocity. In the general field of electromyography, however, a number of different techniques have been developed which allow more detailed and, to some extent, objective and quantitative analysis to be applied to particular aspects of the neuromuscular system (Lenman, 1969).

ACTION POTENTIAL MEASUREMENT

Although the measurement of the mean amplitude of action potentials is of limited usefulness, since the values obtained depend to a large extent on the technique of recording, measurements of mean action potential duration have made it possible to define sets of normal values and establish the range of values to be expected in particular conditions. It can thus be applied as a diagnostic method governed by objectively established criteria. Provided the method of recording is maintained constant, the histogram showing the distribution of action potentials for a given muscle in normal individuals is reasonably consistent, although it is dependent on age (Buchthal et al., 1954). In the diagnosis of disease it is particularly valuable in muscular dystrophy, where the mean action

31

potential duration is short (Buchthal and Pinelli, 1952) (*see* Chapter 10).

Mean action potential duration is determined by measuring photographed action potentials, which can be done most easily if they are displayed in single sweeps of the oscilloscope with a fast time base (not less than 5 msec/cm), so that the action potentials appear relatively spread out. A convenient arrangement is to photograph the traces on slowly moving film with the camera so arranged that the film moves at right angles to the X-axis of the oscilloscope tube. Because it may be difficult to determine the exact onset and termination of a potential, each potential should be recorded several times, and an adequate number, preferably more than twenty, must be photographed and measured (Buchthal *et al.*, 1954). The onset and termination of each potential must be established according to strictly defined criteria, and since the values obtained depend, among other things, on the electrode characteristics, the results can be evaluated only against normal values obtained in the same laboratory. The method is time-consuming and requires meticulous attention to detail, and for this reason has had limited application as a routine method.

AUTOMATIC FREQUENCY ANALYSIS

The mean duration of the action potentials and, more particularly, the proportion of potentials that are polyphasic, are reflected in the frequency analysis of the interference pattern if it is subjected to Fourier analysis.

It is possible to obtain an automatic analysis of the frequency distribution of the electromyogram using a system of tuned circuits, so that the frequency analysis is displayed on the oscilloscope simultaneously with the interference pattern (Richardson, 1951). Using this technique it has been found (Plates 9, 10 and 11) that whereas the dominant frequency in the limb muscles in normal subjects is in the region of 200 c/s, in muscular dystrophy the dominant frequency may be greater than 400 c/s (Walton, 1952). This method, if it is used in association with a loudspeaker, has a certain usefulness in clinical work, as it may assist in interpreting the oscilloscope record and the auditory record in doubtful cases. However, it does not provide the certain and objective information that may be obtained from action potential duration measurement (*see* Chapter 10).

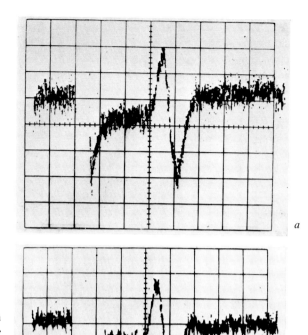

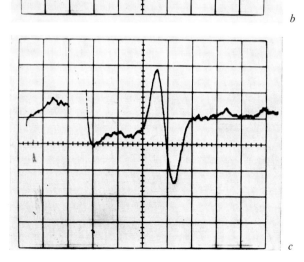

PLATE 1 Nerve action potential (mixed sensory and antidromic motor) evoked from median nerve at elbow of healthy subject following stimulation of the median nerve at the wrist. In trace (*a*) the upper frequency response of the pre-amplifier is 40,000 c/s; in trace (*b*) it has been reduced to 10,000 c/s and in trace (*c*) to 1,000 c/s. It is evident that reducing the band width of the system causes a marked reduction in the background noise but only a small reduction in the size of the evoked potential. In each record the squares of the graticule represent 1 msec on the horizontal axis and 10 μV on the vertical axis.

a

b

c

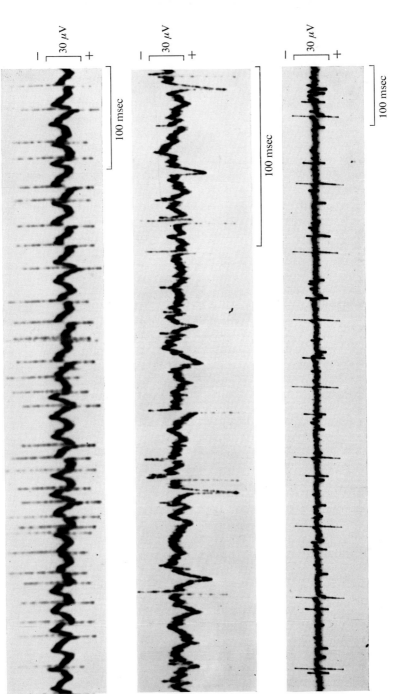

PLATE 2 Abnormal insertion activity and fibrillation potentials in partially denervated muscle. Trace (a) shows high frequency discharges evoked by electrode movement. Traces (b) and (c) illustrate fibrillation. In trace (b) it is evident that the potentials have an initial positive phase. In trace (c) fibrillation potentials are seen to be occurring at a frequency of about 10/sec.

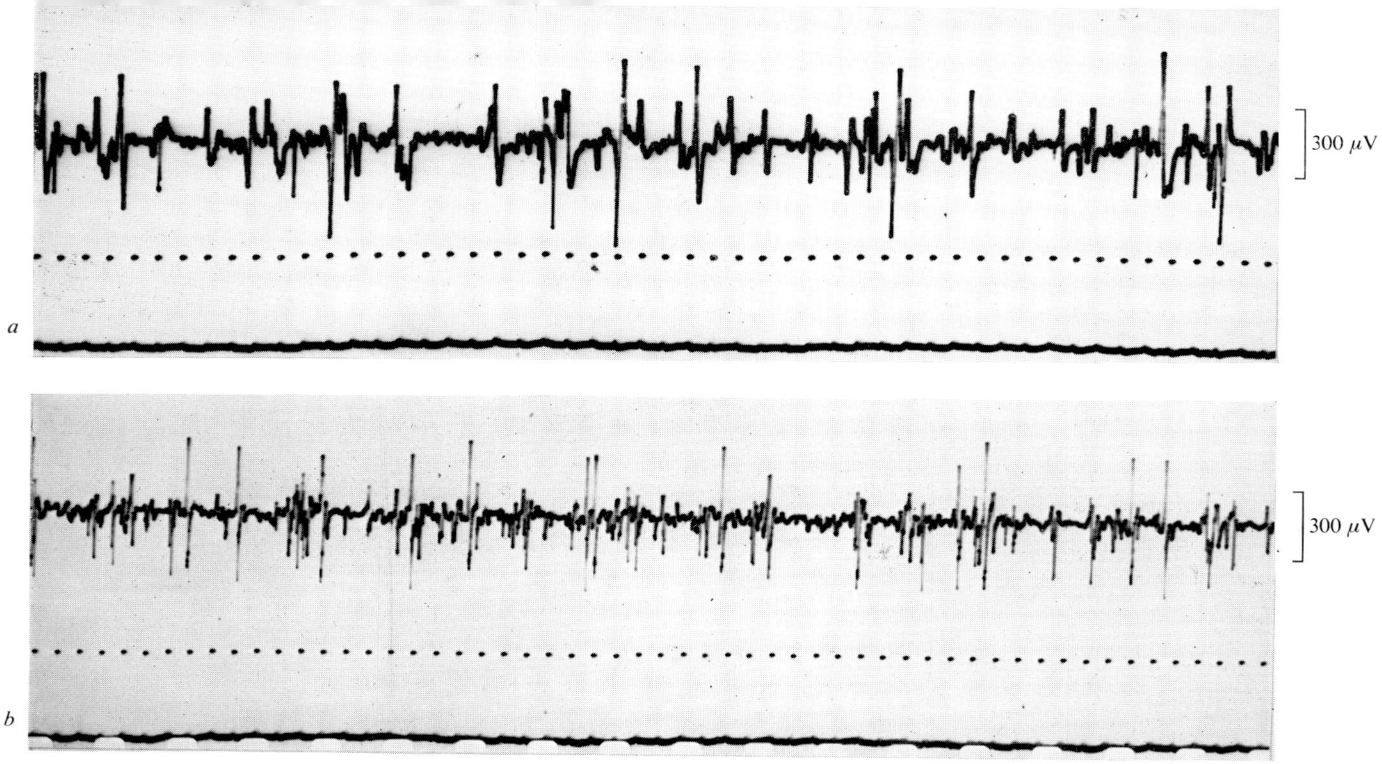

PLATE 3 Normal motor unit potentials recorded from (a) the first dorsal interosseus muscle, and (b) the frontalis muscle. The potentials recorded from the facial muscles are of relatively short duration compared with those recorded in the limb muscles. Time scale 10 msec.

300 μV

300 μV

a

b

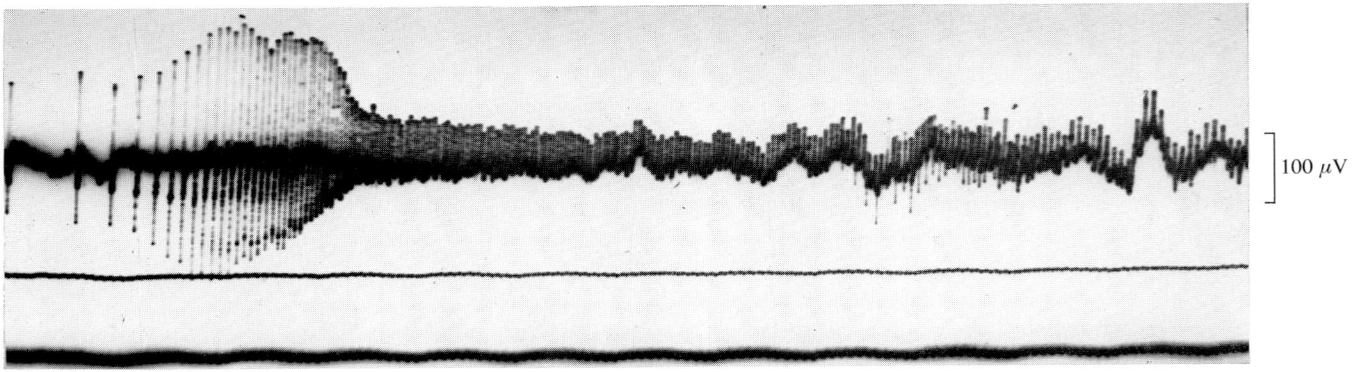

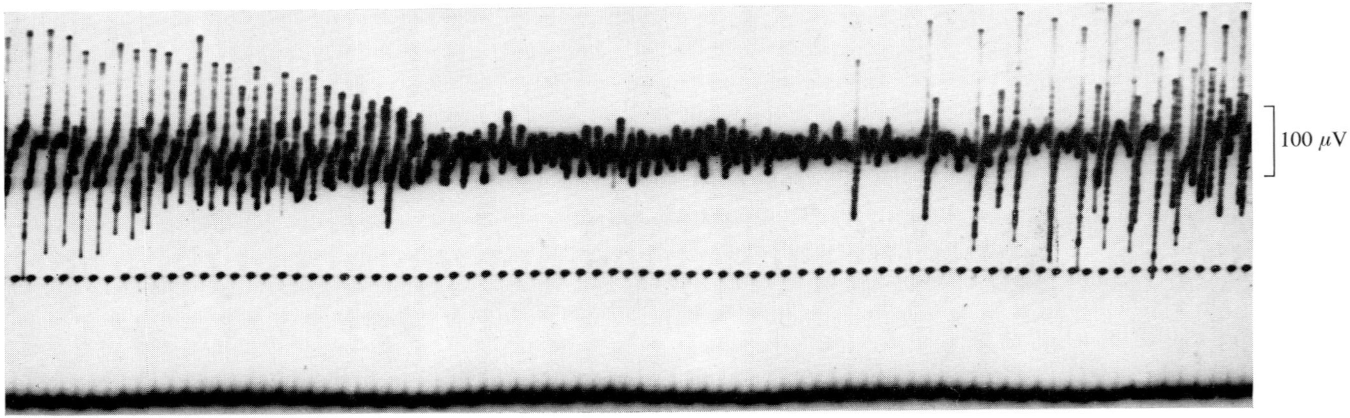

PLATE 4 (above) and 5 (below) Myotonic discharges evoked by electrode movement in patient with myotonia congenita (Thomsen's disease). Time scale 10 msec.

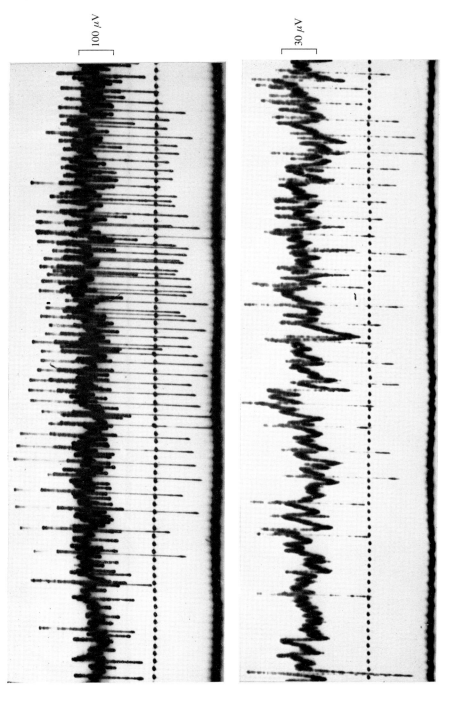

100 μV

30 μV

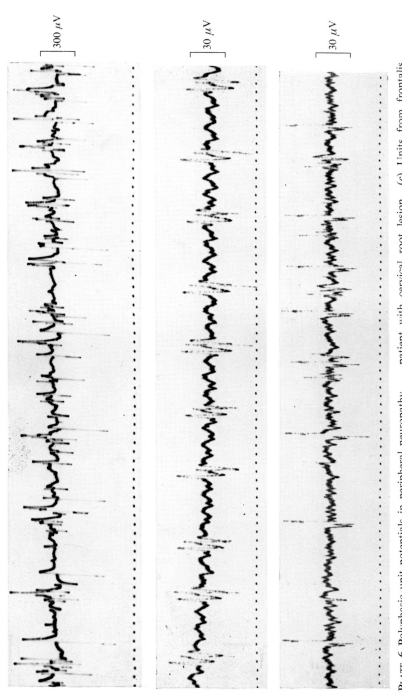

PLATE 6 Polyphasic unit potentials in peripheral neuropathy. (a) Units from deltoid muscle of a patient with peripheral neuritis. (b) Units in partially denervated deltoid muscle of patient with cervical root lesion. (c) Units from frontalis muscle of patient with Bell's palsy. Time scale 10 msec.

PLATE 7A High amplitude long duration potentials recorded from patient with motor neurone disease. Time scale 10 msec.

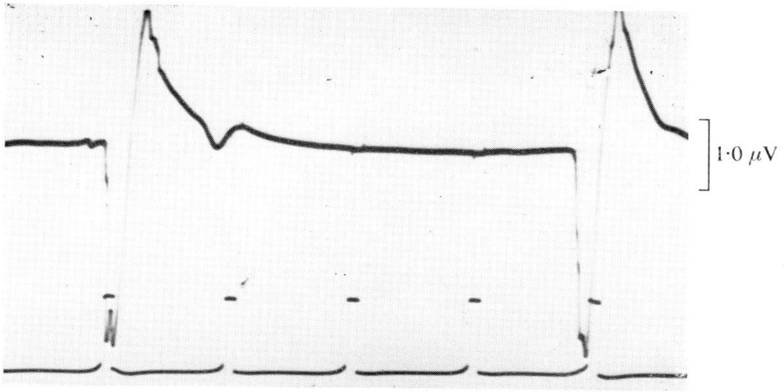

1·0 μV

PLATE 7B (below) Polyphasic units recorded from quadriceps muscle of a patient with muscular dystrophy. Time scale 10 msec.

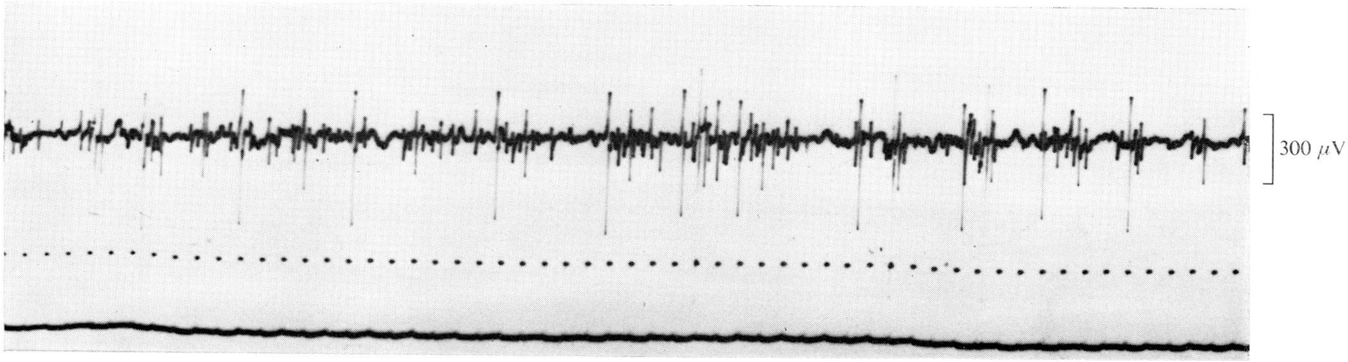

300 μV

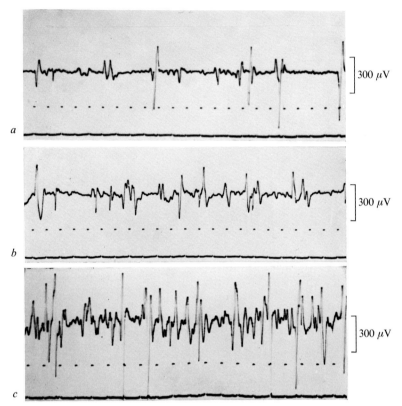

a

$300 \, \mu V$

b

$300 \, \mu V$

c

$300 \, \mu V$

PLATE 8A Motor unit action potentials from normal dorsal interosseus muscle during progressively more powerful contractions. In the interference pattern (c) individual units can no longer be clearly distinguished. Time scale 10 msec.

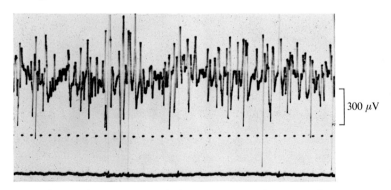

$300 \, \mu V$

PLATE 8B Interference pattern during strong muscular contraction. Time scale 10 msec.

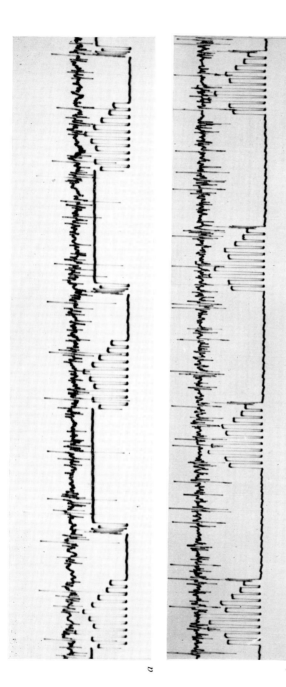

PLATE 9 Frequency analysis of EMG from quadriceps muscle of patient with muscular dystrophy (*a*) and a normal frontalis muscle (*b*). The short duration potentials recorded from the facial muscles may give rise to a high frequency pattern in the automatic analysis similar to that seen in the limb muscles in muscular dystrophy.

a

b

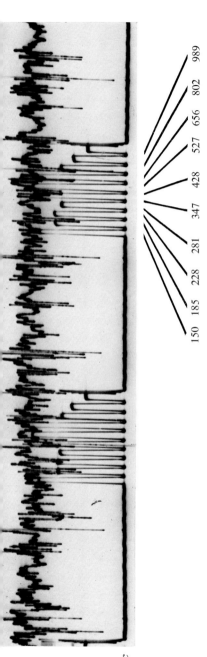

150   185   228   281   347   428   527   656   802   989

PLATES 10, 11 Frequency analysis of EMG from normal muscle (a) and from dystrophic muscle during weak (b), and strong (c), contraction.

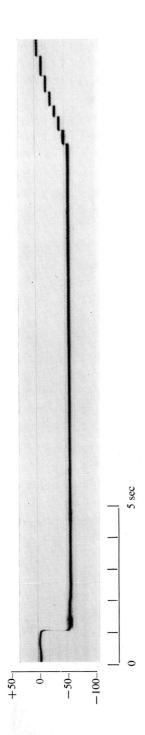

PLATE 12 Resting membrane potential recorded from muscle fibre of healthy mouse. The abrupt fall in potential signals the entry of the microelectrode into the muscle fibre. The amplitude of the potential is measured by applying a voltage (in 10 mv steps) from a calibrator to return the trace to the base line.

SYNCHRONISATION AND MOTOR UNIT TERRITORY

Under normal circumstances, if two concentric electrodes are inserted into different parts of a muscle and the action potentials recorded by them are displayed on two independent channels on an oscilloscope screen, it is seen that there is no consistent time relationship between the motor unit potentials recorded from different parts of the muscle. In patients with disease affecting the anterior horn cells of the spinal cord, such as poliomyelitis, simultaneously occurring potentials can be recorded from electrodes situated far apart in the same muscle (Buchthal and Clemmeson, 1943).

The explanation for this apparent synchronisation is uncertain (*see* Chapter 8). If two electrodes were to record from different parts of an enlarged motor unit this could account for synchronisation (Denny-Brown, 1949), and measurements of the territory occupied by single motor units have shown that in anterior horn cell disease the motor units are considerably enlarged (Erminio *et al.*, 1959). This enlargement of units, however, is probably not adequate wholly to account for synchronisation and it is possible that in anterior horn cell disease there is also some form of interaction between spinal neurones (Buchthal and Madsen, 1950; Simpson, 1962 and 1966).

Multi-electrode electrodes have thrown considerable light on motor unit structure both in health and disease. The multi-electrode used is a stainless steel electrode, which contains twelve independent leads that record from separate points along its length. Using this electrode one can measure how far apart along the needle track it is possible to record potentials identifiable as coming from the same motor unit and, hence, map out the distribution of units within the muscle (Buchthal *et al.*, 1959). From these studies, it is clear that in peripheral nerve lesions the increase in motor unit territory is smaller than in anterior horn cell disease (Erminio *et al.*, 1959), whereas in many cases of muscular dystrophy and polymyositis the territory is reduced (Buchthal *et al.*, 1960).

INTEGRATION AND SPIKE FREQUENCY MEASUREMENT

If the electromyogram is recorded through surface electrodes and the mean voltage of the action potentials is determined either by planimetry or by electronic integration, it can be shown that the integrated mean voltage during graded voluntary contractions has a linear relationship to the isometric tension of the muscle (Lippold, 1952). It is possible to plot the slope of mean voltage against isometric tension during voluntary contractions, and the muscles most easily studied in this way are the biceps and triceps in the upper limbs and the triceps surae in the lower limbs. Since the ratio of voltage to tension is linear, and since isometric tension is related to the number of motor units activated, the integrated electrical activity is a measure of motor unit activity. The curve relating voltage to tension is, thus, a measure of the efficiency of a muscle in terms of the number of motor units activated for a given level of contraction.

The slope of this curve is altered during fatigue in a manner which suggests that when a muscle is fatigued more motor units are required to maintain a given tension (Edwards and Lippold, 1956). Likewise, many patients with muscular dystrophy show a similar alteration in the slope of the voltage tension curve, suggesting that the ability of dystrophic motor units to develop tension is reduced (Lenman, 1959). The change which occurs in the voltage tension relationship during fatigue may be modified if there is neuromuscular block, as in myasthenia, or abnormal muscle stiffness, as may occur in rheumatoid arthritis (Lenman, 1966; Lenman and Potter, 1966).

The relationship between motor unit activity and tension in voluntary contractions may also be studied by counting the number of spikes in the interference pattern when this is recorded with concentric electrodes in the muscle. When this is done by counting the spikes in a photographed record it is liable to error, since there is a large element of subjective assessment in deciding whether small changes in potential should be designated as spikes. This difficulty can be overcome by electronic counting using a system which registers all changes in phase above a certain voltage. The demonstration of a high spike frequency at a standard tension by this method is a reliable means of indentifying dystrophic muscle (Willison, 1964; Rose and Willison, 1967; Dowling et al., 1968; Willison, 1968) (see also Chapter 10).

REFRACTORY PERIOD MEASUREMENT

If a muscle is stimulated through a bipolar electrode, inserted distal to the innervation zone, to avoid stimulating the intramuscular nerves, the action potentials of quite small groups of muscle fibres can be recorded with electrodes inserted proximally in the muscle.

After a single shock the muscle is refractory to further stimuli for a short interval of time, and this refractory period has been defined as the shortest interval after the first or conditioning stimulus when a second or test stimulus will evoke a response (Lucas, 1910). The first part of the refractory period is known as the absolute refractory when the muscle cannot be excited by any stimulus, no matter what its strength. This is followed by the relative refractory period when a sufficiently strong stimulus may be effective. The absolute refractory period depends on the recovery time of the muscle fibre after it has been depolarised (Buchthal and Engbaek, 1963), and must therefore be related to the membrane properties of the muscle fibres. It is difficult to measure accurately because there is considerable scatter between the measurements for different fibres, and it is essential that the groups of fibres activated with each set of stimuli should be as small as possible and care is necessary to avoid excessive stimulus artefact (Buchthal et al., 1955; see also Chapter 4). The normal range for refractory period in healthy muscle has been found to lie between 2·2 and 4·6 msec (Farmer et al., 1960).

The clinical interest of refractory period measurement is that the refractory period of dystrophic muscle is shorter than that of healthy muscle (see Chapter 10), and it may also be abnormally short in clinically healthy carriers of muscular dystrophy (Farmer et al., 1959; Caruso and Buchthal, 1965).

INTRACELLULAR ELECTRODE STUDIES
The earliest studies of the electrophysiological properties of single muscle cells were made on the isolated sartorious muscle of the frog, when the potential difference across the cell membrane was measured by inserting a glass micropipette electrode into the fibre (Graham and Gerard, 1946; Ling and Gerard, 1949). Since that time the method has been intensively applied to the study of amphibian, avian, and mammalian muscle and a great deal has been learned regarding the fundamental properties of muscle fibres. More recently the technique has been applied to the study of diseased muscle, both in the experimental animal and the human subject (Johns, 1964). The technique is not at present suitable for routine clinical use but the information which has so far been obtained from it is of fundamental interest.

The muscle fibre membrane has a potential difference across it of about 90 mV, with some variation between different species, the outside positive and the inside negative. This potential difference is maintained by differences in the concentrations of positive and negative ions on either side of the membrane and by the selective permeability of the membrane to different ions. Thus, sodium exists in high concentration in the extracellular fluid whereas potassium exists in high concentration within the cell. The membrane in the resting state is permeable to potassium and chloride but relatively impermeable to sodium. Energy is required to maintain the different concentrations of sodium and potassium outside and within the cell and this energy is provided by a metabolic process, sometimes referred to as the 'sodium pump', which enables sodium to move out of the fibre while potassium moves in.

The potential across the cell membrane is known as the resting membrane potential and this is maintained by a variety of interacting factors. It is clear from studying the effect of altering the concentrations in the extracellular fluid (Hodgkin and Horowicz, 1959) that it follows closely the K concentration gradient which can be expressed quantitatively by the Nernst equation

$$E_k = \frac{RT}{F} \log_e \frac{(K_i)}{(K_0)}$$

(Where E_k is the K equilibrium potential (K_i) and (K_0) the potassium concentrations inside and outside the cell and R, T and F as the gas constant, the absolute temperature and the Faraday constant.)

When a muscle is activated the polarity across the membrane is reversed so that an action potential occurs. This depolarisation is brought about by a sudden alteration in membrane permeability so that it becomes permeable to sodium which moves into the cell. This is followed by an outflow of potassium which restores the resting condition and a final phase in which the membrane permeabilities return to their original state. In some way the action potential triggers off the contractile process within the muscle fibre. The action potential originates in the end-plate zone where the action of acetyl choline gives rise to the end-plate potential, this initiates the depolarisation which is propagated along the fibre membrane. When the muscle is quiescent, small potentials are continuously appearing in a random manner at the end-plate zone. These have an amplitude of 1 to 2 mV, are known as miniature end-plate potentials, and are probably due to the action on the end-plate membrane of small quantities or quanta of acetyl choline which are continuously released from the nerve ending (Castillo and Katz, 1956). The resting membrane potential of a muscle fibre can be measured by inserting a microelectrode. As soon as the electrode enters the cell the tip becomes negative and an abrupt fall in potential of 80–90 mV is registered (Plate 12). If the muscle is now activated by stimulating its motor nerve or by stimulating the fibre directly, an action potential will be recorded. In denervated muscle action potentials will occur spontaneously. If the microelectrode is inserted in the end-plate zone, miniature end-plate potentials may be recorded.

If a second electrode is inserted into a muscle fibre and a current passed through it, the physical properties of the membrane can be measured by observing the changes in the membrane potential. Important characteristics which can be studied in this way are the membrane resistance and capacity, the product of which gives the membrane time constant. Another use of a second electrode is to apply chemicals such as acetyl choline electrophoretically to particular sites on the membrane.

Microelectrode studies may be carried out either *in vivo* or on excised muscle mounted in a chamber containing suitable bathing fluid. In the study of muscle disease both methods have been applied and each has its advantages. Isolated muscle can be transilluminated and kept stationary so that it is much simpler to insert more than a single electrode. With muscle *in situ* the environment is more nearly physiological, and the difficulty in stimulating the muscle through a second electrode can be partially overcome by passing a stimulus through the single recording electrode, using a Wheatstone bridge arrangement to compensate for the artefact produced (Araki and Otani, 1955). While it is most satisfactory to insert the electrode into muscle which has been exposed by incising the skin, this can be avoided by enclosing the electrode within an outer steel cannula which is used to penetrate the skin (Beranek, 1964). If this method is used the electrode capacitance is considerably increased and it is necessary to use an amplifier which compensates for this.

When measurements are made of the membrane potential the usual practice is to measure the potential between the microelectrode and a reference electrode at earth potential in contact with the extracellular fluid and connected to one input lead of the amplifier

(Fig. 3.1). The potential may be measured by applying an equal voltage in opposite sense from a calibrator in series with the reference electrode. Important precautions which should be taken while recording are to monitor the electrode resistance and tip potential. If the electrode becomes blocked as it enters the muscle a potential may develop across the tip, which can cause serious errors (Adrian, 1956).

Observations which are relevant to neuromuscular disease have been made on denervated muscle, on myopathic muscle, and on muscle affected by myotonia, periodic paralysis, and myasthenia gravis.

Information concerning single muscle fibres in denervated muscle is, at present, entirely derived from animal experiments. In the frog

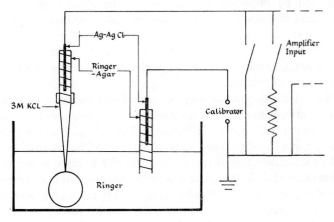

FIGURE 3.1 Circuit arrangement for recording resting membrane potential of muscle fibre.

there are important differences in membrane characteristics following denervation, such as an increased membrane resistance and a lowered threshold to electrical stimulation (Nicholls, 1956). In mammals, most workers have reported a lowered resting membrane potential in denervated muscle; the explanation for this is not certain but it may be related to changes in membrane conductance (Ware, et al., 1954; Lüllmann and Pracht, 1957; Thesleff, 1963; Lenman, 1965).

In muscular dystrophy in the mouse the resting membrane potential is lowered (Kleeman *et al.*, 1961; Lenman, 1963; McComas and Mossawy, 1964) and a low resting potential has been recorded in excised intercostal muscle in human muscular dystrophy (Ludin, 1968). In human dystrophia myotonica a lowered resting potential has been found both in excised muscle (Hofmann *et al.*, 1966), and *in situ* in exposed muscle (McComas and Mrożek, 1968). In dystrophic muscle the resting potential has been shown to follow the potassium equilibration potential, and it is possible that the low resting potentials in muscular dystrophy may be related to a lowered content of intracellular potassium (Horvath and Proctor, 1960).

A low resting membrane potential is one possible explanation for the abnormal excitability of muscle in myotonia (*see* Chapters 2 and 10), since muscle fibres would be expected to depolarise more readily if the resting potential were close to the depolarisation threshold. This hypothesis, however, has not been supported by studies of myotonic muscle where the dystrophic features which are characteristic of dystrophia myotonica are absent. Thus, in the myotonic goat the resting potential has been found to be normal (Bryant, 1962). In myotonia congenita, although only a few cases have been studied, and there are differences between the results obtained in different centres, normal resting potentials have also been recorded (Norris, 1962; Riecker *et al.*, 1964; McComas and Mrożek, 1968).

In familial periodic paralysis (*see* Chapter 10) where the extracellular potassium is low, and where it has been postulated that the intracellular potassium may be high, a raised resting membrane potential during attacks might be an expected finding. However, in the small number of cases studied, the contrary has been the case, since the resting potential has been normal or below normal (Shy *et al.*, 1961; Creutzfeldt *et al.*, 1963). In hyperkalaemic periodic paralysis, on the other hand, where the extracellular potassium is markedly raised, the expected finding of a low resting potential has been confirmed (Creutzfeldt *et al.*, 1963; McComas *et al.*, 1968).

In myasthenia gravis (*see* Chapter 11) observations have been made on excised intercostal muscles. In an early study, the resting potential was found to be normal and in the end-plate zone miniature end-plate potentials were seen to occur infrequently, although they appeared to be of normal amplitude (Dahlbäck *et al.*, 1961).

Subsequent work in the same laboratory showed that the average frequency of miniature end-plate potentials was no different from that of normal muscle, but that their amplitude was reduced to about one fifth of normal, a size at which they could readily be lost in the background noise of the recording system. This small size was not due to altered sensitivity of the muscle fibre membrane to acetyl choline, because the membrane responded normally to applied cholinergic drugs. It was concluded that the defect in myasthenia gravis is likely to be pre-junctional and is related to a reduced amount of acetyl choline in each of the transmitter particles or quanta which pass from the nerve endings to the muscle membrane (Elmqvist *et al.*, 1964).

Hofmann *et al.* (1967) and Elmqvist and Lambert (1968) have studied excised intercostal muscle from patients with muscular weakness similar to that occurring in the myasthenic syndrome, which may be associated with bronchial carcinoma (*see* Chapter 11). The results in the two studies differ in certain respects but, in each, miniature end-plate potentials were recorded which were of normal or nearly normal amplitude and the end-plate potential following a single nerve impulse tended to be of low amplitude. These findings indicate that the sensitivity of the muscle fibre to acetyl choline is normal, but that a reduced number of transmitter particles are released by the nerve impulse. In the patient described by Elmqvist and Lambert, repetitive stimulation of the nerve fibre at 40/sec resulted in an increase in amplitude of the end-plate potentials. In this patient the neuromuscular block showed some resemblance to the block which may be produced experimentally by botulinus toxin or by high magnesium concentration.

The evidence at present available from microelectrode electrode studies is in favour of a pre-junctional block in both myasthenia gravis and the myasthenic syndrome associated with carcinoma. However, the nature of the prejunctional defect is different in the two conditions. In myasthenia the quanta of transmitter which are released appear to contain a reduced quantity of acetylcholine. In the myasthenic syndrome, on the other hand, the nerve impulse seems unable to bring about the release of an adequate number of quanta of transmitter substance.

It is clear from this brief review that intracellular studies have thrown considerable light on the mechanism underlying some of the defects in neuromuscular disease. Unlike some of the quantitative methods referred to earlier, which have an obvious clinical application, they may have little immediate relevance to clinical diagnosis. It is likely, however, that future work along these lines will further clarify many of the important questions which at present remain unanswered.

4
The Measurement of Nerve Conduction Velocity

Conduction velocity in a peripheral nerve was first measured by Helmholtz (1850), initially in the frog and later in man. He recorded the difference in mechanical latency of a muscle on a myograph after stimulating two points of a nerve in succession. In later studies Piper (1908) used the evoked potential in muscle to measure the time of arrival of nerve impulses. The clinical value of this procedure did not become evident until the Second World War when experimental work on animals showed that, following nerve crush or suture, the conduction velocity in a regenerating nerve fibre is slowed (Berry *et al.*, 1944). This was subsequently confirmed in human peripheral nerves (Hodes *et al.*, 1948) and, following this, the method has been widely applied to the study of peripheral neuropathy and nerve compression syndromes.

Originally, studies were confined to measuring motor nerve conduction velocity and the technique employed was to stimulate the motor nerve at two points along its course recording an evoked potential from the muscle it supplied. Subtraction of the shorter from the longer latency gave the conduction time along a segment of the nerve, and if the length of this was measured the conduction velocity could be calculated. The conduction velocity could not be derived from a single latency, because part of the latency between nerve and muscle is due to the delay which occurs at the neuromuscular junction. Nevertheless, the terminal latency following a stimulus applied to the distal end of a motor nerve gives useful information in the study of syndromes where there is local pressure in a distal part of the nerve, as may occur in compression of the median nerve in the carpal tunnel (Simpson, 1956).

Although nerve action potentials are of much smaller amplitude than muscle potentials, they can be recorded quite readily if suitable electrodes are placed on the skin overlying the nerve (Dawson and Scott, 1949). Such potentials can be evoked by applying a stimulus

42

to a mixed nerve, in which case the action potential may be partly derived from stimulation of sensory fibres and partly from antidromic activation of motor fibres. Action potentials derived from stimulation of sensory nerves alone can be evoked by electrical stimulation of the fingers through ring electrodes (Dawson, 1956), or by application of a tactile stimulus such as tapping of a nail (Sears, 1959). The study of sensory nerve action potentials has been shown to be of considerable value in peripheral nerve disorders (Gilliatt and Sears, 1958).

Although conduction velocity and latency are the most generally useful parameters in respect of peripheral nerve function, the characteristics of the evoked potentials are also important. With muscle potentials the duration of the potential is of interest, because slowing of conduction in a few fibres of the motor nerve may result in late activation of part of the muscle and the potential may be both prolonged and polyphasic. When nerve action potentials are recorded temporal dispersion due to slowed conduction in some of the fibres may lead to a significant decrease in amplitude.

When carried out in association with electromyography the study of motor and sensory nerve conduction provides a useful technique for the recognition and accurate localisation of peripheral nerve pathology. A useful supplementary method is to record potentials which can be evoked reflexly by stimulation of a peripheral nerve. By this means the reflex time can be measured and this gives an indication of the conduction time in the proximal segments of a peripheral nerve. In certain circumstances it is also possible by this method to estimate the excitability of a reflex and obtain information regarding central excitability in the spinal cord.

APPARATUS AND TECHNIQUE

ELECTRODES

Evoked potentials in a muscle can be recorded either with concentric needle electrodes or with surface electrodes. Concentric electrodes have the advantage that they can be inserted accurately into a particular muscle and the action potentials have a sharp take off which can be more readily identified than the curved origin of the potential recorded with surface electrodes (Simpson, 1964). On the other hand, they require adequate sterilisation and are painful to insert, which restricts their use in children and in patients who require repeated examinations. They are particularly valuable when it is necessary to study conduction along a particular terminal branch of a peripheral nerve, such as for example, the deep branch of the ulnar nerve in the hand. Surface electrodes may be small discs, about 1 cm in diameter made of stainless steel or silver which are covered with electrode jelly and applied to the skin. The usual practice is for one electrode to be applied over the belly of the muscle, the other over the tendon. A useful development has been the introduction of clip-on electrodes which consist of a clasp of stainless-steel wire with two sharpened points which spring together to clip on to the skin (Copland and Davies, 1964). These are simple and relatively painless to apply and are particularly useful in situations such as the face, where firm adhesion of surface electrodes may be difficult to achieve.

For recording nerve action potentials, silver disc electrodes held in perspex about 3 cm apart are satisfactory. Where the evoked potentials are small they can be recorded with more certainty with unipolar electrodes inserted close to the nerve. This may be done by inserting two needles about 3 cm apart with the tips close to the nerve (Gilliatt et al., 1961). Alternatively, a single recording electrode may be placed close to the nerve and the potential recorded against an indifferent electrode placed several centimetres from the nerve, but approximately equidistant from the stimulating cathode (Buchthal and Rosenfalck, 1966).

For stimulating peripheral nerves, silver discs covered with lint and soaked in saline are suitable. For bipolar stimulation, two electrodes held in perspex 3 cm apart may be used and are arranged so that the cathode, which is the active electrode, is closest to the recording electrodes. For unipolar stimulation, a single cathode made of a silver disc covered in lint is placed over the nerve; the anode may be a plate of zinc attached proximally (in the case of motor nerve stimulation) to the limb.

For stimulating digital nerves to evoke sensory potentials thin strips of silver covered in lint soaked in saline are generally suitable (Dawson, 1956).

STIMULATORS

While a capacitor discharge can provide a perfectly adequate stimulus for exciting a nerve, a stimulator capable of delivering square wave pulses of known amplitude and duration is commonly employed.

The stimulator should be designed so that pulses of relatively short duration will deliver enough current to the tissue to stimulate all the rapidly conducting fibres comprised in the nerve. The brevity of the pulse is important because, in the first place, long duration pulses may activate neighbouring muscles and, second, brief pulses are less likely to excite pain fibres than long duration pulses, which also may give rise to repetitive firing (Fig. 4.1). Generally speaking,

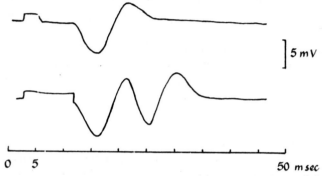

FIGURE 4.1. Effect of increasing duration of stimulus. Evoked potential recorded from abductor digiti minimi after stimulation of the ulnar nerve at the elbow with 3·0 msec pulse (upper trace) and 10 msec pulse (lower trace). Repetitive firing could account for the later potential in the lower trace.

pulse durations of between 10 and 300 μsec are satisfactory and a maximum output of at least 200 V is desirable.

In order to minimise stimulus artefact it is necessary that the output of the stimulator should be isolated from earth. This can readily be achieved by delivering the stimulus through an isolating transformer or through a radiofrequency isolating unit (Donaldson, 1958; *see also* below). In addition to providing the stimulus, the stimulator should give out a pre-pulse to trigger the oscilloscope sweep. This pre-pulse should precede the stimulus by a short delay so that the whole stimulus artefact appears on the oscilloscope trace (Simpson, 1964).

RECORDING APPARATUS

The requirements for the amplification and display of evoked potentials are similar to those stated elsewhere for electromyography. Since evoked muscle action potentials are generally of several millivolts in amplitude, the requirements in respect of amplifier gain and noise level are not abnormally exacting when motor nerve conduction velocity is measured. On the other hand, evoked nerve action potentials may be only a few microvolts in amplitude so that for sensory nerve conduction studies high gain and low noise levels are important. For this purpose it is desirable that the system should have a sensitivity such that signals of 10 μV may be displayed to have an amplitude of not less than 1 cm. The inherent noise level of the system should be as low as possible, and it is important to have the means of reducing this further by adjusting the frequency response to one or two kc/s (*see* Chapter 2).

Where very small signals are to be displayed there are several methods of recording potentials that are of about the same amplitude as the overall noise level. One is to photograph a series of superimposed recurrent sweeps; when this is done a regularly recurring signal may be distinguished from the random fluctuations of the background. A further step is to use an averaging computer which adds the recurring signal electronically by a process which does not affect the noise level. A less elaborate method which has been used to increase the signal-to-noise ratio is to interpose a step-up transformer between the recording electrodes and the input of the amplifier (Buchthal and Rosenfalck, 1965).

The arrangements for oscilloscope display and photography of evoked potentials are similar to those employed for electromyography. A useful refinement in apparatus adapted for nerve conduction studies is to use an oscilloscope which has a storage tube. This allows the stored trace to be viewed and measured before a permanent photographic record is made.

TECHNIQUE

Conduction velocity measurements have the merit that they are quantitative observations which depend neither on the co-operation of the patient nor the subjective impressions of the observer. Nevertheless, there are many possible sources of error and the details of technique are particularly important if serious errors are to be avoided.

Accurate measurement is not possible when the record is obscured by artefact. Movement artefact is generally fairly easily avoided if the limb is positioned carefully in a comfortable posture, and if the nerves are stimulated by brief pulses which do not excite muscle. Fifty cycle interference from the mains supply is much less of a difficulty with modern apparatus, particularly when balanced amplifiers are used. It may still, however, cause difficulty if the patient is not properly earthed, if there are loose connections, if the input leads are too long and not properly screened, and if the laboratory is positioned close to some important source of interference. When high gains are employed, as in recording sensory nerve potentials, particular care needs to be taken to reduce mains interference.

An important source of interference is derived from the fact that the stimulator is delivering a pulse of perhaps several hundreds of volts to the tissue, while the recording apparatus is arranged so as to record signals of a few millivolts or less. The stimulus artefact is liable to be particularly large if the stimulus is passed through an earth electrode common both to stimulator and amplifier. For this reason, a transformer is frequently placed between the output stage of the stimulator and the patient to isolate the stimulator from earth. There may, however, still be difficulty unless precautions are taken because the capacitance between the transformer secondary and ground may allow transient currents to flow between the stimulus site and the earth electrode. This capacitance leak to earth can give rise to stimulus artefact and also in certain circumstances to spurious stimulation at the earth electrode. The use of a radio frequency isolating unit can avoid this difficulty, but is itself capable of producing interference through transmission of radio frequency energy. If an isolating transformer is used the capacitative escape to earth can be reduced by using a double transformer screen. The primary screen is connected to earth and the secondary screen may be floating or can be connected to the patient through an additional electrode. This arrangement is useful when a bipolar needle electrode is used to stimulate muscle, as in refractory period measurement (*see* Chapter 3) when the screen can be connected to the shaft of the stimulating electrode. Under these circumstances the capacitance between the stimulator and earth is replaced by the capacitance of the screen, and the capacitative current can flow to the extra electrode and not to the earth electrode. The use of transistor circuits in stimulator design may also be helpful since if the stimulator can be built to a small size the overall capacitance to earth can be kept low. Another important technical factor is to record with an amplifier with a high rejection ratio, and with an input impedance of sufficient magnitude that the rejection ratio is maintained even if recording electrodes of high impedance are employed (Buchthal *et al.*, 1955; Guld, 1960 and 1961; Neilson, 1962).

In the practical setting up of the procedure the application and positioning of the electrodes are important. Stimulus artefact is particularly liable to give trouble when the stimulating and recording electrodes are situated in close proximity, and will be greater the more widely the recording electrodes are spaced apart. The skin should be carefully prepared under both the recording and stimulating electrodes to reduce the skin resistance. This may be done by cleaning the skin first with ether to dissolve the surface grease and then rubbing the skin gently with an abrasive such as fine sandpaper. Stimulus artefact is less likely to be troublesome, the lower the source impedance provided by the recording electrodes and the underlying tissues. A brief stimulating pulse will give rise to a smaller artefact than a pulse of long duration, and a brief pulse is more likely to pass sufficient current into the tissue to excite the nerve if the skin resistance under the stimulating electrodes has been reduced to a low level. An important precaution, which materially affects the size of the stimulus artefact, is that the earth plate which connects the patient to ground should be placed so as to lie between the stimulating and recording electrodes.

If a nerve is stimulated with a weak stimulus and then the intensity of the stimulus is progressively increased, it is frequently found that the latency of the evoked potential shortens as the stimulus intensity increases (Dawson, 1956). It is clear that a weak stimulus will not necessarily activate all the most rapidly conducting fibres in the nerve, and in order to measure nerve conduction velocity it is necessary to be certain that the stimulus is strong enough to do this. This is achieved by using a stimulus that is at least 30 per cent greater than a supramaximal stimulus. A supramaximal stimulus is obtained by placing the stimulating electrode over the nerve and first applying a series of pulses of moderate intensity. The position of the electrode is then adjusted until further movement no longer increases the size of the action potential (Downie, 1964). When the best stimulating site has been found, the strength of the stimulus is increased until increasing the stimulus further has no effect on the size of the evoked potential. The voltage required to provide a supramaximal stimulus depends on a number of factors including the pulse duration, the output impedance of the stimulator and the impedance of the tissue. In practice, with short pulses voltages in excess of 200 V may need to be employed. If the stimulus current is measured, it is found that a current in excess of 20 mA may be necessary to provide a supramaximal stimulus (Buchthal and Rosenfalck, 1966).

To calculate a motor nerve conduction velocity it is necessary to obtain two latencies, one from a proximal and one from a distal site along the nerve. Subtraction of the distal from the proximal latency gives the conduction time along the segment of nerve between the two stimulating sites, and if the length of this segment of nerve is measured the conduction velocity can be calculated. The distal latency between the distal stimulating electrode and the recording electrode in the muscle includes the time taken for the impulse to

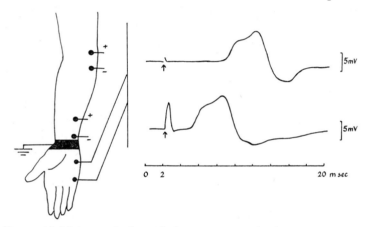

FIGURE 4.2 Motor conduction velocity measurement in the ulnar nerve of a healthy subject. Evoked potentials are obtained from abductor digiti minimi after stimulation of the ulnar nerve at elbow and wrist. If the distance between the two stimulating cathodes is measured and divided by the difference between the two latencies the conduction velocity from elbow to wrist is calculated. In this record the stimulus occurs 2·0 msec after the sweep is triggered. The earth electrode is placed between the stimulating and recording electrodes to lessen the stimulus artefact.

cross the neuromuscular junction and, hence, does not give a true indication of conduction velocity along the nerve. The time of arrival of the nerve impulse at the muscle is taken as the moment when the evoked potential leaves the baseline. If this method is to be free from error it is important that the evoked potential obtained from stimulating the nerve at proximal and distal sites should be similar in shape, so that comparable points can be taken as representing the take-off in each case (Fig. 4.2).

If a high gain is necessary to record an evoked potential from a muscle, a small negative potential is sometimes observed immediately preceding the compound action potential. This potential may be a nerve action potential derived from nerve fibres underlying the recording electrode, and it may give rise to confusion if it is regarded as the first phase of the compound action potential from the muscle (Simpson, 1964). It is particularly liable to cause error if the evoked potential derived from nerve stimulation at one site requires a higher recording sensitivity than the action potential evoked by stimulation at a second site.

In the measurement of sensory nerve conduction the evoked potentials are recorded from nerve, and conduction velocity can be calculated after measurement of the latency between the evoked potential and a single stimulus. The evoked potential, however, is very much smaller than a muscle potential and the amplitude may not greatly exceed the noise level of the recording apparatus. The shape of the evoked potential is partially dependent on the method of recording. In general, nerve action potentials recorded in the human subject differ from the potentials recorded from isolated nerves where the initial deflection is a negative one caused by the wave of depolarisation passing under the recording electrode. Under clinical conditions, the situation is more complicated because the potentials recorded by electrodes external to the nerve depend on the laws determining the propagation of an electrical field within a volume conductor (Lorente de No, 1947; Dawson and Scott, 1949). Because of this, the initial deflection is a positive one. With monopolar recording using a single electrode close to the nerve and a remote indifferent electrode, the potential is triphasic with an initial positive phase. With bipolar recording, using two electrodes close to nerve it may have two, three, or four phases dependent on the distance apart of the recording electrodes (Buchthal and Rosenfalck, 1966). Measurements of conducting latency give different values dependent on whether the initial positive phase of the potential or the later negative peak is taken as the point of measurement, since these intervals become farther apart the farther the recording electrodes are separated from the stimulating electrodes. This is probably because the duration of the action potential increases the farther the recording site is removed from the stimulus, due to dispersion of impulses carried by fast and slow conducting fibres (Dawson, 1956). Measurement of the latency to the positive peak gives the more accurate conduction time (Buchthal and Rosenfalck, 1966), but is not always possible since this part of the potential is frequently small or cannot be recorded, and this is particularly likely to be the case in peripheral nerve lesions when the sensory potential may be greatly reduced in size, or absent (Gilliatt and Sears, 1958). For this reason, measurements are frequently made to the peak of the negative deflection. When this is done during bipolar recording, allowance can be made for the fact that the negative peak occurs later than the arrival of the impulse at the first recording electrode, by measuring the conduction distance to the mid-point between the two recording electrodes (Downie, 1964).

Nerve conduction velocity is dependent on temperature and it is therefore important to measure conduction latencies under conditions of adequate temperature control.

Johnson and Olsen (1960) report a change in conduction velocity of about 5 per cent for every deg C change in temperature. In motor nerve conduction velocity measurements, where velocity is calculated after subtraction of two latencies, the error is to some extent avoidable since a change in the proximal latency may be to some extent compensated by a corresponding change in the distal latency. However, where there is peripheral wasting there may be a temperature gradient along the limb (Simpson, 1964), and where nerve action potentials are used in measurement the error is no longer a systematic one. Strict temperature control involves the measurement of subcutaneous temperatures with inserted thermistors. This has the disadvantage that additional skin punctures are necessary and there are problems in connection with sterilisation. However, if the limb to be examined is carefully warmed before each set of measurements, and is covered with blankets during the test, and if measurements are not made when the skin temperature is below 30 deg C errors due to changes in temperature are unlikely to be serious.

MOTOR NERVE CONDUCTION

Motor nerve conduction velocity can be readily measured in the median, ulnar, common peroneal, and posterior tibial nerves, and in these the technique is widely used as a routine diagnostic test. Methods have also been developed for measuring conduction in the radial (Gassel and Diamantopoules, 1964), sciatic (Gassel and Trojaborg, 1964), and femoral nerves (Gassel, 1963). Terminal latencies are also of value in distal compression neuropathies and can readily be determined in the major peripheral nerves of the upper and lower limbs. The facial nerve is readily accessible in its distal segment and the terminal latency between the angle of the jaw and either orbicularis oris, or the frontalis muscle, can be determined (see Chapter 9).

Average values for motor nerve conduction velocity in different peripheral nerves have now been established in many different laboratories and, in general, the findings are consistent. They do, however, differ in some degree according to the details of recording technique, and it is therefore appropriate for each laboratory to establish a normal range based on its own average values (Table 4.1). Generally, conduction velocity in the upper limbs is more rapid than in the lower; thus, in one series the mean for the ulnar nerve supplying abductor digiti minimi was 56·2, S.D. 4·6, and range 49·0 to 65·6 m/sec, whereas the mean for the common peroneal nerve to extensor digitorum brevis was 49·7, S.D. 7·1 and range 35·6 to 63·5 m/sec (Thomas et al., 1959). Below the age of three, nerve conduction velocity is relatively slow and it reaches the normal mean at about the age of five (Thomas and Lambert, 1960). In adult life there is a slow decline in conduction velocity with advancing years (Wagman and Lesse, 1952) (see also Chapters 7 and 8).

SENSORY NERVE CONDUCTION
Sensory nerve conduction can be readily measured in the median and ulnar nerves by using ring electrodes applied over the fingers (Fig. 4.3). It is common practice to apply these electrodes over the distal phalanx and over the base of the proximal phalanx. However, in the case of the median nerve there may be an advantage in using the base of the second phalanx for the proximal electrode, since the skin over the dorsal aspect of the first phalanx of the first two fingers may be supplied by the radial nerve. While it is usual to apply the stimuli to the ring electrodes and record the orthodromic sensory potential, it is also possible to stimulate the nerve proximally and record antidromic sensory potentials from the ring electrodes over the finger. Where it is only possible to record small action potentials by this method, it is sometimes helpful to apply the stimulus simultaneously to two or more digits. If this is done, the stimulus is applied to the fingers from separate stimulators: if the same stimulator is used, it is not possible to deliver the same current to the individual fingers on account of the differences in impedance (Buchthal and Rosenfalck, 1966).

In the ulnar nerve, evoked potentials can be recorded from different sites on the nerve to as high as the axilla. With the median nerve potentials can also be recorded from the nerve at and above the elbow. The recording of orthodromic sensory potentials is more difficult in the radial nerve, but in this nerve satisfactory potentials can be recorded by antidromic stimulation.

In the lower limb, sensory potentials can be evoked in the posterior tibial nerve by applying stimuli with ring electrodes. In this situation,

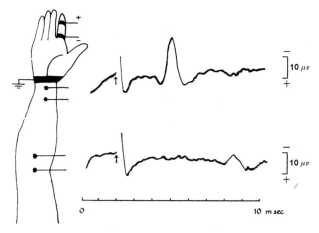

FIGURE 4.3 Sensory nerve action potentials evoked from the median nerve of a healthy subject at the elbow and wrist after stimulation of the index finger with ring electrodes. The potential recorded at the wrist is triphasic but the potential at the elbow is comparatively small and the initial positive phase is less easily identified.

however, it is difficult to record evoked potentials without using subcutaneous electrodes. Nerve action potentials can also be obtained from this nerve by stimulating the posterior tibial nerve at the ankle and recording proximally from the medial popliteal nerve. When this is done, however, not only are the sensory nerve fibres stimulated, but the motor nerves are also activated so that antidromic impulses pass up them. The action potential recorded from the nerve is therefore derived from impulses conducted along both sensory and motor nerve fibres.

Since the mixed orthodromic sensory and antidromic motor nerve action potential is often of larger amplitude and more easily recorded than the pure sensory potential, this technique is a useful one and is readily applied to the median and ulnar nerves. It may also be used to measure conduction velocity in the common peroneal nerves which are not readily accessible to direct sensory stimulation. Here

TABLE 4.1

Nerve Conduction Measurements in Control Population of Adult Subjects without Evidence of Neuromuscular Disease
(Lenman, 1969)

Peripheral nerve	Number of nerves	Range metres/sec	Mean metres/sec	SD
Peroneal (motor) knee to ankle	49	42·1–63·5	52·1	4·9
Posterior tibial (motor) knee to ankle	30	39·8–66·9	49·9	5·2
Ulnar (motor) elbow to wrist	47	46·5–72·6	59·9	5·7
Median (motor) elbow to wrist	45	46·1–72·1	56·9	5·8
Ulnar (sensory) finger to wrist	52	41·7–59·4	49·4	4·7
Ulnar (sensory) finger to elbow	38	45·3–60·2	55·2	3·5
Median (sensory) finger to wrist	48	36·4–65·4	52·0	6·1
Median (sensory) finger to elbow	36	42·4–61·7	55·9	5·8
		msec	msec	
H reflex latency	32	26·5–34·0	29·8	1·8

again, recording with surface electrodes is difficult and it is more satisfactory to use a needle electrode in close apposition to the nerve fibre (Gilliatt *et al.*, 1961).

The normal values for conduction velocity in sensory nerves are of the same order of magnitude as those for motor nerves (Table 4.1) although the fastest conducting sensory nerves may conduct at a slightly faster rate than the most rapidly conducting motor nerves (Dawson, 1956).

REFLEX EVOKED POTENTIALS

If a peripheral nerve is stimulated and an evoked potential is recorded from the muscle it supplies, it is sometimes possible to record a second potential which occurs later than the initial response. Whereas the latency of the initial response decreases the nearer the stimulating electrode is brought to the muscle, with the second potential the reverse may be the case so that the latency increases

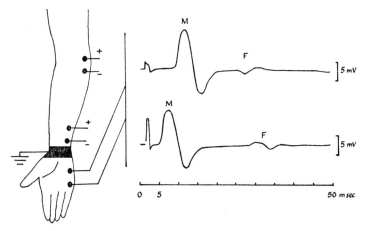

FIGURE 4.4 F wave recorded after stimulation of the ulnar nerve at the elbow and wrist. The later potential has a longer latency following stimulation at the wrist than following stimulation at the elbow.

as the stimulus approaches the muscle. This indicates that the stimulus of the late potential must first travel proximally along the nerve for a certain distance before travelling distally to activate the muscle. In some instances the latency of the late potential is sufficient for the impulse to have travelled proximally as far as the spinal cord to activate a spinal reflex.

One such late potential is readily evoked after stimulation of the ulnar and median nerves, provided strong stimuli are used. It has a latency of up to about 30 msec and its amplitude is substantially smaller than the directly evoked potential or M wave. This late potential can be evoked after stimulation of the majority of peripheral nerves in the upper or lower limbs, and it has been termed the F wave (Fig. 4.4) by Magladery and McDougall (1950) who considered that it represented a spinal reflex. It has subsequently been shown that it can still be evoked in animals after division of the posterior roots and it probably represents the discharge of spinal motor neurones after antidromic activation (McLeod and Wray, 1966).

If the posterior tibial nerve is stimulated a late potential can be

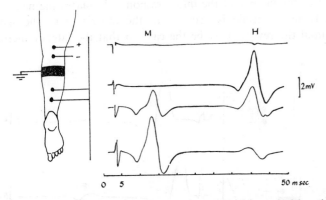

FIGURE 4.5 The H reflex. The four traces show potentials evoked by stimulation of the medial popliteal nerve with pulses of increasing magnitude (top trace shows weakest stimulus). The later potential or H wave is a low threshold response which is maximal when evoked by a stimulus too weak to evoke the M wave or directly evoked muscle response. As the M wave increases in amplitude the H wave diminishes.

evoked from the triceps surae muscle which has different characteristics. It is a low threshold potential which appears before the stimulus is adequate to evoke the M wave, and after reaching a maximum amplitude it decreases in size as the stimulus intensity is increased, so that with a supramaximal stimulus it is usually absent (Fig. 4.5). This potential was first described by Hoffmann (1918) and is known as the H wave. Its latency (Table 4.1) is comparable to that of the F wave, but unlike the F wave it cannot be elicited from stimulation of nerves other than the posterior tibial without some form of facilitation. It has been shown to represent a spinal reflex (Magladery et al., 1951) and is, in fact, the electrical homologue of the ankle jerk, and like the ankle jerk represents a monosynaptic reflex.

Both the F wave and the H wave can be used to study the conduction velocity in the central segments of peripheral nerves and in this respect are of interest in the study of peripheral neuropathy. The H wave, however, has an added interest because it is a reflex response, and the ease by which it may be obtained depends, among other things, on the excitability of the motor neurone pool in the spinal cord. Thus, in the presence of spasticity the F reflex can quite readily be evoked by stimulating other peripheral nerves apart from the posterior tibial nerve. The level of reflex excitability can be studied quantitatively by using paired stimuli to evoke the F reflex in a manner analogous to the determination of refractory period (Magaldery *et al.*, 1952). If this is done, it is found that during a period from 10 to about 100 msec after the stimulus which evokes the H wave it is not possible to evoke a second response, and thereafter there is a period of up to several seconds when the excitability of the reflex is abnormal. In patients with spasticity, flaccid paralysis, and Parkinsonian rigidity this recovery cycle is altered (Diamantopoulos and Olsen, 1967; Olsen and Diamantopoulos, 1967; Yap, 1967). The determination of the recovery cycle is, at present, subject to many technical limitations, and it is particularly liable to be modified by peripheral factors such as incomplete relaxation; moreover, the tremor of Parkinson's disease may impose a serious difficulty. For this reason the clinical value of the H reflex in the analysis of reflex excitability is not yet fully established (Lenman, 1969).

A relatively uncommon late potential may occasionally be evoked in the small muscles of the hand in patients with peripheral nerve lesions. Its latency is shorter than that of the F wave and not long enough to allow for passage of the impulse to and from the spinal cord. It is probably an axon reflex due to nerve fibre branching (Fullerton and Gilliatt, 1965).

5
Electrical Stimulation: Intensity-Duration Curves

Electrical stimulation as an adjunct to diagnosis of peripheral nerve lesions has been practised for over a century, and the first coherent accounts of its utility in human cases were given by Erb (1868; 1869; 1883). At that date accurate quantitative measurements of excitability were not practicable, and diagnostic importance was attached to qualitative changes, such as sluggishness of contraction and reversal of the polar effects of galvanic current, in identifying what was described as the 'reaction of degeneration'. The older literature is very extensive, and it is interesting to observe how often advances were made more by improvements in technology than physiological or clinical insight. A most readable and interesting historical survey is given by Sidney Licht, 1961.

Electrodiagnostic stimulation is not commonly undertaken on a scale which permits direct comparison and assessment of various methods, and it is important to appreciate the principles and limitations involved. We are only concerned, here, with percutaneous stimulation of human tissues, which is essentially less precise than the procedures that can be carried out experimentally on exposed tissues. A valuable modern account of stimulation in general, not confined to human tissues or to electrical methods, is given by Kay (1966).

In 1883, Erb described the distinction, by stimulation through unbroken skin, of normal innervated human muscle from muscle where motor nerve supply had been fairly recently, i.e. within months, destroyed, and this important radical distinction can be done by a variety of methods, some quite simple. In practice, however, it is often important to achieve a refinement of the distinction between normal and totally denervated muscle, in that it is desirable to distinguish, if possible, states of partial innervation where the muscle is a complex of mixed normal and denervated tissue. The natural history of nerve regeneration is such that recovery

58

is necessarily a slow process, involving complete growth of new axons from injury site to periphery. It is usual for muscle to re-innervate in sections, gradually building up enough units to reveal clinically detectable contraction; some time before this stage is reached, certain regions of the muscle are in fact re-innervated, though too weak to produce movement, and their detection is of great value in diagnosis and prognosis.

A great many techniques of electrodiagnosis have been devised and employed to a greater or less extent, and are to be found in the literature cited, but it should be said that the best and most reliable information is only to be obtained by processes which approximate to careful research.

All methods are based on producing depolarisation at the membrane of nerve or muscle fibre by means of electrical changes artificially applied to the surface of the body, and while the characteristics of the electric pulses at the surface may nowadays be very accurately determined, it is impossible to describe with precision the magnitude and time course of events at the membrane surface consequent upon the applied pulse.

Indeed, when one considers the complex electrical properties of the skin and tissue layers which intervene between the region of application and the point of depolarisation, it is surprising that so much useful and repeatable quantitative information can be obtained from percutaneous stimulation. If the tissue elements behaved as true resistances, obeying Ohm's Law, the problem would be intricate enough; but they do not, and because the equivalent electrical circuit of tissues is both complex and variable, we must be content with approximate and sometimes empirical observations attested by clinical trial. Recent mathematical treatments of the impedance of human tissue with percutaneous stimulation of the type used in diagnosis have been published by Stephens (1956; 1960).

Earlier methods, intended to formulate a single numerical 'index' of excitability (Cluzet, 1913; Lewis Jones, 1913; Lapique, 1926; and others) proved unsatisfactory in practice.

GALVANIC-FARADIC TEST

A test which has survived since Erb's description is that widely known as the galvanic-faradic test, dependent on the observation that a long-lasting stimulus (galvanic shock) will excite both nerve and muscle whereas a short stimulus, as from the secondary winding of a faradic coil will excite nerve but not muscle. Therefore, according to the test, if muscle responds to the faradic shocks it must be at least partially innervated; if it responds only to the galvanic shock, it is denervated.

The galvanic-faradic test is obsolete and can be misleading. In an analysis of 10,000 galvanic-faradic tests on peripheral nerve injuries occurring during the 1939–45 War, it has been shown that the test has only a 50 per cent chance of being correct, and has virtually no value in prognosis (Ritchie, 1954).

INTENSITY-DURATION CURVES

PRINCIPLES

The technique which has so far proved most satisfactory in large-scale clinical trials is the recording of the intensity-duration relationship of applied electrical stimuli. Originally shown by Adrian (1917) to be applicable to human nerve injury, modern electronic technology has developed instruments of precision and convenience in practical use. The principle of their operation is simple and fundamental, that a short-duration shock will depolarise at a high intensity, and a long-lasting shock at a much lower, or threshold, strength. The relationship between the strength of a stimulus and its duration in time, for constant response of an excitable tissue, gives an accurate measure of the excitability of that tissue, and is referred to as the intensity-duration curve.

This type of relationship, wherein a physical or chemical change can be produced by high-intensity short-duration effect and by low-level longer time action is not confined to excitable tissues; it applies, to give a household example, in the 'blowing' of a protective fuse which, indefinitely intact below a threshold (its rated value as a fuse), will melt or rupture either on sustained small overload, or gross transient overload, or at various combinations of intensity-duration in between.

Instruments to produce the necessary wave-forms at appropriately calibrated durations and intensities are available commercially, and have been a fruitful field for inventors. The original human intensity-duration curves produced by Adrian (1917) were recorded from a mechanical pendulum of considerable mass which, when released, successively knocked over two contacts where separation controlled the duration of the shock; this ingenious apparatus was too cumbersome and slow for routine clinical use, and, in fact, the utility of the method had to await modern electronic pulse generators.

STIMULATOR IMPEDANCE EFFECT

Some explanation is required of the expressions high-impedance (constant current) and low-impedance (constant voltage) as applied to stimulators.

In order that the intensity calibration may remain correct under varying circumstances of application such as size of electrodes, resistance of skin, and impedance of deeper tissues, it is customary to design the output circuit of stimulators in one of two ways. The first way is to include in series with the electrodes a resistance that is very high (ten or twenty times the highest likely inter-electrode resistance). This high internal resistance is usually obtained electronically, and results in the current flow between the electrodes being independent of the electrode and inter-electrode impedance. Such high-impedance generators are calibrated in current flow, usually 0–100 mA, and are termed 'constant-current' stimulators, an ambiguous expression meaning that the current as registered on the output calibration dial or meter will be delivered at that value regardless of variations in electrodes and tissues.

The second basic variation of design has, in parallel with the electrodes, a resistance many times lower than any likely to be encountered between the output terminals by external connection of electrodes and tissues; again, this low resistance effect is devised electronically by feed-back methods. As inter-electrode resistances have a negligible effect on the voltage appearing at the terminals (because they do not significantly reduce by shunting what is already a very low resistance), such low-impedance instruments are termed 'constant-voltage', meaning that the voltage is stabilised with respect to the output calibration. The output is variable from 0 to 150, or 200 V.

In both cases, the pulse duration control provides a variety of pulse lengths ranging from 0·1 msec up to 300 msec; as this very wide range can only satisfactorily be recorded on a logarithmic scale, the intervals are usually provided in the series 1, 3, 10, and so on.

There are technical and physiological complications which have only relatively recently been appreciated, in that the actual quantitative figures obtained depend on the internal impedance of the apparatus (Stephens, 1956; Brennand, 1959). There are also practical clinical considerations in that the theoretically more precise high-impedance generator frequently used in animal experiment is not so suitable for human application as the less technically elegant low-impedance design which is better tolerated by the human subject (Stephens, 1961; Ritchie, 1954; Wynn Parry, 1964).

TECHNIQUES

The production of precision and calibration-stable stimulators has simplified electrode technique, which in most modern practice has become established as the use of one large 'indifferent' electrode (i.e. one which serves as the electrical return and plays no direct part in excitation) and an active electrode, moveable and of suitable size and shape for the region to be examined, usually about 1–2 cm in diameter, though smaller ones may be used for small muscles such as those of the hand. It is good practice to connect the large indifferent electrode to a sound electrical earth—most machines are connected internally this way, for the modern stimulator, carelessly used, is capable of delivering a pulse which can be dangerous—and to arrange polarity so that the active small electrode is negative, during the pulse ON period, in relation to earth. Stainless steel, with a saline-soaked pad cover, is the most satisfactory material for electrodes, and obviates the corrosion commonly found with other metals. Excitation using two small electrodes placed longitudinally with respect to a muscle, is valuable in some cases as an alternative to monopolar stimulation (Wynn Parry, 1953).

At each duration setting of the time-calibrated control, it is necessary to determine the intensity, in volts or milliamperes according to the type of stimulator, at which minimal detectable response occurs; this intensity figure, for each duration, is the variable from which the curve is plotted.

Although many arrangements have been devised to detail the muscle twitch which results from a pulse above threshold, by mechanical means, in practice, palpation and inspection show a surprisingly high degree of repeatability, and it has not been found necessary to go to additional complication.

At the same time, the operator should provide himself with the optimal adjuncts in respect of good lighting and a comfortable, warm position for the subject.

A complete system involves the recording of action potentials consequent upon stimulation, and the method has been used by

Doupe (1943) and Thomas and Morton (1963). The additional complication is considerable, because the action potentials have to be detected very shortly after the very much greater stimulus artefact produced by the stimulus shock. The problem arises in connection with nerve conduction velocity measurements, but the stimulus is short and can readily be isolated from earth; the long pulses essential for an intensity-duration curve on denervated muscle present much more difficulty. Thomas and Morton employed a special transistorised isolated stimulator, and concluded that the intensity-duration curves recorded, with some technical difficulty, by this dual technique of electrical stimulation/electrical recording corresponded to those obtained by inspection of mechanical response, and point out that further work, together with some technical improvement, is necessary if the results are to be significantly more informative.

It is important to realise that when working with human subjects where disability or injury may involve pain on movement, speed and comfort of the diagnostic process is an essential factor; a prolonged and painful recording technique, however scientifically precise, may yield indifferent results or be inapplicable to a number of cases. This consideration will be discussed more fully in connection with the practical choice of stimulators for percutaneous human use.

It was at one time usual to include, in texts of Electrodiagnosis, diagrams of the so-called 'motor points' of muscles; these are the surface regions, often quite sharply defined, below which the motor nerve breaks up into its terminal distribution to the muscle, or where the terminal nerve elements are concentrated. The motor point is, in effect, the skin region wherefrom innervated muscle is most accessible to percutaneous excitation at the lowest intensity. Although the motor point is an anatomical entity, it is not exactly located from one patient to another, and of course it is non-existent in denervated muscle; in practice, with modern stimulators having a variable and calibrated control of output, it is a simple and speedy matter to identify the motor point by trial.

It is more important to possess a thorough knowledge of the innervation order of the muscles supplied by a given nerve; some nerves are represented in Fig. 7.1 in connection with conduction velocity measurements, and a useful complete set of diagrams together with photographs of clinical tests for individual muscle action is to be found in *MRC War Memorandum* (1942) No. 7. This information is of value in that muscles re-innervate, if regeneration occurs in a definite anatomical order dependent on the length of axon path to be reconstituted, and observations on a proximally-innervated muscle may be repeated at a later date on one more distal; they may not appear at all in the latter if the progress of re-innervation ceases.

CHRONAXIE; CURVE ASSESSMENT

Because of the complex impedance of tissue, the actual figures recorded on an intensity-duration curve depend not only on the excitability of the nerve or muscle, which is what one wants to know, but to some extent on the built-in properties of the stimulator.

Figure 5.4 represents a family of I-D curves from the same muscle,

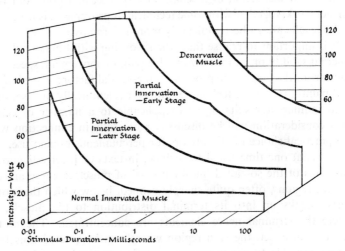

FIGURE 5.1 Generalised diagram of intensity-duration curves recorded with low impedance, constant voltage type of stimulator (500 Ω output; five-point curves). The 'kinks' or discontinuities corresponding to the dual excitability of partially denervated muscle states alter in position on the graph as reinnervation progresses (Ritchie, 1952). (Reproduced by courtesy of *Physiotherapy*.)

with the same electrodes, taken with a stimulator where internal impedance could be varied from 10 Ω (constant voltage, low-impedance) to 1 MΩ (constant current, high-impedance).

Two points of great importance emerge. In the first place, the curves are of the same shape, but they are displaced relative to each other on both the time and the intensity axis. It will be shown that, in practice, shape is more valuable as a diagnostic criterion than absolute numerical value, so that this complication—the variation of the plotted curve with the stimulator, used on the same tissue—is less serious than might appear. But, second, any attempt to express the curve by one single numerical figure is useless, unless associated with the internal impedance of the stimulator with which the measurement was made. The most widely known index is that called 'chronaxie' by Lapique (1926), which is, by definition, the time required for a stimulus of twice the threshold (rheobase) strength to be effective for constant response. The rheobase, theoretically the smallest effective intensity required to provoke response if allowed to continue indefinitely, can, in practice, be determined by rectangular pulses of about 1 msec duration from a constant-voltage generator, or 10 msec duration for a constant-current stimulator. These figures refer to normal muscle innervated through an intact motor nerve; freshly denervated muscle requires durations several hundred times longer to determine the rheobase.

Having established the rheobase for a given detectable response, the voltage is doubled, and the time for which such a pulse must last, to produce the same response, is the chronaxie.

Although various 'chronaximeters' have been used, the index is best calculated from the complete curve, as in Fig. 5.4.

Referring to the three curves taken from normal muscle, it is apparent that the chronaxie figure varies from 0·03 to 0·2 msec by variation of the stimulator impedance alone, and this on the same tissue with the readings made within a few seconds of each other. The apparent simplicity of attempting to express 'excitability' by a single figure index is defeated by the sophistication of electronic techniques in producing stabilised stimulators of different types. While it remains true that with a particular stimulator specification chronaxie figures will be comparable, they will not tally with results obtained from another and different instrument, and the transform of chronaxie in relation to output impedance is far more complex and much less informative than the recording of the complete curve.

In respect of denervated muscle, the chronaxie variation with stimulator impedance is much less, for reasons connected with the longer stimuli used for denervated muscle.

But the most important objection to the use of any single numerical index stems from the fact that, so far, the most valuable information from clinical intensity-duration curves comes from discontinuities in the curves, which do not obey simple mathematical rules, and cannot be expressed by chronaxie, or indeed manifested other than by inspection of the complete curve. It is fortunate for the value of the method that the human capability of perceiving such discontinuities, 'kinks', or double curves, when presented in graphic form is high.

STIMULATOR SPECIFICATION

With regard to the choice of stimulators, there are several conflicting requirements. A critical survey of the relationship between the output impedance and performance of stimulators has been produced by Stephens (1960). He makes the point that, in general, low impedance constant-voltage stimulators are better tolerated by the

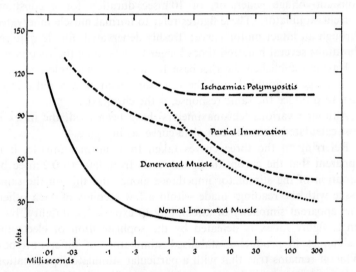

FIGURE 5.2 Characteristic intensity-duration curves recorded with a low-impedance stimulator. The rise of threshold voltage necessary for excitation as duration is diminished is typical of denervated muscle; contrast with the 'flat' part of the normal muscle curve, which rises only when the shock duration is below one millisecond.

A very high rheobase with a flat type of long-duration plot is suggestive of ischaemia or polymyositis, but is not of itself diagnostic.

patient than constant-current types; this is supported after extensive clinical trial by Wynn Parry (1953) and Ritchie (1954), and was accepted by a Sub-Committee of the Medical Research Council which, after reviewing the available clinical evidence, came to the conclusion that, 'the voltage calibrated generator is considered to be an adequate instrument for general use for electrodiagnosis of neuromuscular disorders'.

The MRC Sub-Committee published a specification (1958) of electrical requirements which can be summarised as follows:

(a) *Pulse duration*—10 pulse widths shall be available as follows: 300, 100, 30, 10, 3, 1, 0·3, 0·1, 0·03, 0·01 msec. Pulse width accuracy shall be ±5 per cent or 1 μsec, whichever is the greater.

(b) *Pulse repetition* frequencies shall be 0·5, 5, and 50 pulses/second.

(c) *Pulse amplitude* shall be 200 V maximum for all pulses. An amplified control in conjunction with a calibrating system shall be employed to set the output to the maximum value of 200 V.

(d) *Output control*—the delivered output shall not differ from the indicated output by more than 10 per cent for all pulses and repetition frequencies, including switching transients. An output dial, directly calibrated in volts, shall be employed in order to provide a greater effective scale length than the size of meter commonly employed.

(e) *Wave form*—this shall be essentially flat-topped for all pulses. Amplitude droop shall not exceed 10 per cent on the 300 msec, and 5 per cent on the remaining pulses. Rise and decay times shall be negligible compared with pulse width. In the case of the 0·01 msec pulse, permissible rise and decay times are 0·001 msec. Leading and trailing edges shall have no more than a single overshoot which shall not exceed 10 per cent of amplitude.

(f) *Output impedance*—shall not exceed 500 Ω at any point on the scale.

(g) *Audible monitoring*—there shall be an optional audible monitoring signal synchronised with the pulses.

(h) *Safety precautions*—one of the patient terminals shall be connected to earth and the case. Dangerous potentials shall be excluded from the patient's circuit in the event of valve or component failure.

This specification is adequate, not ideal; it was devised in order that figures produced should be comparable in different clinical testing centres, and the technological development of high-power transistors has made it possible to improve upon the performance specified, while at the same time simplifying the equipment. But, whatever the content of the 'black box' producing the stimuli, an inferior specification will not suffice for satisfactory diagnostic work.

In practice, it appears advantageous to detect muscle 'twitches' at slow repetition rates around one a second rather than the sustained tetanic type of contraction produced by the faradic coil; the tetanising facility is nevertheless retained in modern stimulators and has occasional use, provided that the operator appreciates the basic limitation that if 50 pulses/second are required to produce tetanic contraction, then each pulse should be 10 msec duration or less.

Wynn Parry stresses that discomfort during test is not only undesirable *per se*, particularly in children or apprehensive patients, but is liable to give misleading results through 'tensioning' of the muscles in anticipation of pain.

Nevertheless, Stephens's analysis points out that diagnostic efficiency is somewhat sacrificed by the use of very low-impedance stimulators, which tend to produce a very low threshold, and mask, in composite curves from partially innervated muscles, the very discontinuities of curvature which are the significant features of the test. Stephens remarks that Giovine (1957) reports the detection of discontinuities in normal muscle, particularly when cold, whereas neither Ritchie nor Wynn Parry has ever reported this; and it is possible that Giovine's use of a high impedance instrument would account for this anomaly.

In summary, it is probable that the low-impedance stimulator has limitations in discontinuity detection, and is thereby somewhat less effective diagnostically than the constant-current type; but it is certain that many patients are intolerant of the constant-current pulses and that curves cannot be recorded at all in such cases. Particularly where electrodes have to be moved, or are liable to be displayed (and the first circumstance applies to most clinical electro-diagnosis), the low-impedance voltage-calibrated generator has practical advantages. These considerations hold only for the recording of intensity-duration curves with rectangular pulses for diagnostic purposes, and are not applicable to therapeutic stimulation or the use of triangular pulses for diagnostic purposes.

There is, of course, no objection to the employment of both types of instrument on the same subjects, other than the time and complications involved, and it is fair to say that more work requires to be done in this field. Either low or high impedance technique has merit; both can yield valuable diagnostic information, and to pursue the matter further brings their comparison into the realms of combined technical and clinical research. The papers of Wynn Parry (1953; 1961), Ritchie (1948; 1954), Stephens (1956; 1960; 1963; 1966), and Kay (1966), will form a starting point.

NORMAL AND DENERVATED MUSCLE CURVES

Referring once again to Fig. 5.4, it will be noticed that the lower or rheobasic part of the normal innervated muscle curve is flat, and that, with a 250 Ω constant voltage stimulator, no increase in threshold is necessary until the pulse duration drops below 0·3 msec.

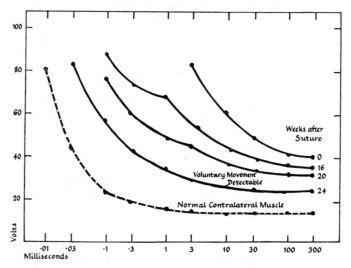

FIGURE 5.3 The electrical course of recovery manifested in the changes in intensity-duration curves (300 Ω stimulator). Curves from Abd. poll. longus muscle after radial nerve suture in upper arm (Ritchie, 1954; case 411). Discontinuities, lowering and flattening of the curves are shown, and the observation times are given; 16 weeks after suture, the first signs of 'electrical' recovery appeared, preceding the earliest detectable voluntary movement by 8 weeks. The curves drawn are selected from weekly records. The 20 week curve, still before voluntary activity, shows the innervation progress from that taken at 16 weeks.

If the threshold is determined at 10 msec, the intensity control left untouched, the pulse duration shortened successively to 3, 1, and 0·3 msec with the response continuing, one may with certainty state that the muscle is being excited via intact motor nerve. Only at pulse durations below 0·1 msec will the intensity control require turning up to cause response to reappear. This is for normal innervated muscle.

Wholly denervated muscle, tested within a reasonable time of denervation, before re-innervation can have begun, and before fibrotic changes have set in, will show a different shape of curve, with the voltage minimal at the 300 msec pulse and rising steadily with shortening of the pulse to 100, 30, 10 msec, and so on. Muscle, depolarised directly, is a less excitable substance than motor nerve.

The distinction between the excitability curves for nerve and muscle is clear-cut; indeed, for a preliminary screening test of innervation or denervation, it would suffice to have an instrument capable of delivering two pulse durations only, one at 100 msec and one at 0·1 or even 1 msec. Normal muscle would respond to both with little or no change of intensity; denervated muscle would contract with the longer pulse and fail to respond to the short one. Such a screening test can, of course, be done with the available stimulators and is useful, though it corresponds to little more than a calibrated galvanic faradic test.

Screening tests of this type with simplified apparatus have been described by Heather and Apostolico (1959) and Bauwens and Richardson (1950), and have merit in selecting subjects for subsequent full intensity-duration curve examination, but they cannot reliably replace the latter.

CLINICAL OBSERVATIONS

It is essential to appreciate the clinical limitations of any method of electrical excitation by percutaneous stimulation. The I-D curves have no concern with neuromuscular pathology; they will attest whether normal, denervated or (in many, but not all, instances) partially innervated/partially denervated muscle underlies the electrodes, but that is the limit of their information yield.

The discrimination between a completely normal and a completely denervated muscle is absolute, and should be 100 per cent reliable if carefully done. Even if the I-D technique were limited to this, it would have real value, because its simplicity, speed of performance, and convenience to the patient allow the examiner to assess a large number of muscles in a short time. Moreover, in cases of functional or hysterical paralysis, a normal I-D curve from the paralysed muscles may immediately solve a problem, for muscles which are inoperative from absence of normal motor unit drive may show no action potentials on electromyography.

But I-D curves do not present shapes characteristic of different types of neuro-muscular disorder as does the electromyogram, and the examiner must infer the pathology and the site of the lesion from basic principles.

The most important conditions made manifest by I-D curve recording are those involving partial innervation, wherein the muscle is a complex made up of normal innervated muscle and completely denervated muscle in varying proportions.

This may come about in a variety of ways: peripheral nerve injury either in the post-traumatic, or, more importantly clinically, in the recovery phase; lower motor neuron damage of any sort, e.g. poliomyelitis and other forms of myelopathy; conditions involving a mixture of neuropathic and myopathic lesions; but not in the myopathies where there is no true denervation.

A complex of innervated/denervated muscle can be identified by 'kink' or discontinuities in the I-D curve, and the relationship of the appearance of these discontinuities to the clinical state has been fully determined and described by Pollock (1944), Newman and Livingston (1947), McKenzie (1949), Ritchie (1954), Wynn Parry (1961), and many other workers. The utility and drawbacks can be summarised fairly simply, because the results of most experienced workers are in very good agreement.

In a small proportion of cases, it is possible to record a complete I-D curve from muscles which the examiner has no reason to suppose are denervated or fibrotic, and in these (1 per cent in Ritchie's series) there is a strong presumption of ischaemic complication. The rheobase may be so high as to be intolerable. Thickening and hardening of the skin will elevate the rheobase, even with good preparation, but the condition is obvious.

Conversion of muscle into non-contractile connective tissue (true atrophy) is a prolonged process, and varies with the anatomical site of the muscle and other conditions such as blood supply. The prevention of such atrophy by therapeutic electrical stimulation as opposed to diagnostic is outside the scope of this book; in brief, there is evidence that intensive therapeutic stimulation can delay but not prevent atrophy, and that improved techniques of stimulation producing the maximal possible contraction could probably improve the position.

In the limb muscles, the period of conversion from denervated muscle to fibrous tissue will occupy many months, and successful re-innervation after surgical intervention may occur up to one or two years, though the residual amount of muscle may be small by that time, and in general, the sooner re-innervation takes place the more satisfactory will be the end result. The facial muscles do not atrophy so rapidly, and contractile muscle may be detected several years after denervation; the reason is not established, but is probably connected with the good blood supply and the continual passive movement of the denervated muscles produced by the underlying muscles of mastication.

The quantitative value of the rheobase is of less significance than the I-D curve shape; the use of low-impedance stimulators masks rheobase changes, and with high-impedance instruments re-innervation is accompanied by a lowering of rheobase. It is doubtful if this minor diagnostic advantage offsets the greater practical utility of the low-impedance type. Where inflammatory conditions occur, as in polymyositis, the rheobase is elevated.

The I-D curve recording technique is sufficiently precise to allow discontinuities to be readily detected by scrutiny of the curve, and serial examinations at intervals are essentially the main use of the procedure; the discontinuity does in fact reveal the simultaneous presence of normal and of denervated muscle, and to some extent their proportions, in a given muscle complex. But in this connection, certain limitations must be borne in mind. As the detectable response to stimulation is the criterion from which the curve is drawn, in some circumstances this may occur late in the process of recovery, or, much more rarely, be unobtainable. The motor units re-innervate in a random fashion, and if the earliest ones to normalise lie in the deep region of a large muscle, or occur scattered throughout the bulk in such a way that they do not, in the early stages, produce an integrated pull on the tendon, then the discontinuity—the appearance of the part of the curve that is due to innervated muscle—may appear late.

In general, the most reliable results will be obtained from the smaller or more superficial muscles.

Again, the detection of re-innervation, as evidenced by discontinuity appearance on serial examination of a muscle hitherto showing only a denervated-type curve, is a guarantee of some degree of recovery, but has no prognostic value as regards ultimate clinical recovery of strength, which depends on the total number of motor units finally re-innervated. The examiner can only say that re-innervation has commenced and cannot predict to what ultimate extent it will proceed. Nevertheless, the assurance of the start of re-innervation is of very great clinical importance, for thereafter there are very few therapeutic measures to be undertaken; and the appearance of discontinuity is a reassurance that any preliminary surgical procedure such as suture, decompression, and the like, has

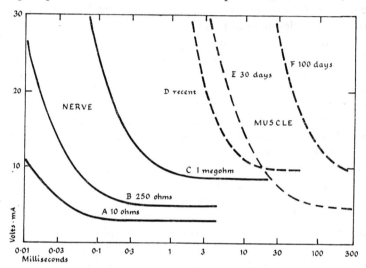

FIGURE 5.4 The effect of stimulator impedance on intensity-duration curves (redrawn from Stephens). The three full-time curves A, B and C were consecutively recorded from the same muscle, altering only the output impedance of the stimulus source. Although the shapes are superimposable, the actual time and intensity values differ; moreover, the chronaxie values (A = 0·03 msec: B = 0·05 msec: C = 0·2 msec) cannot be used to express the curves. A, B and C represent the excitability of human motor nerve, whereby the normal muscle is activated.

The broken curves, D, E and F, are typical of denervated muscle as recorded with a high impedance stimulator (1 MΩ). D represents recently denervated or curarised muscle; E and F show the typical rheobase changes to be expected with a constant-current stimulator, E about 30 days prior to re-innervation, with a lowered rheobase, and F at 100 days after denervation which is complete. No nerve excitability component appears, and curves DEF represent the excitability of human muscle alone.

The vertical scales have been adjusted so that voltage figures (low impedance) and current figures (high impedance) coincide; in ABC the stimulator impedances are given.

been effective at least to the extent of allowing regeneration. The degree of clinical strength recovery thereafter is a matter of time.

There is general agreement that I-D curve discontinuities in re-innervating muscle appear, in favourable circumstances, several weeks before the smallest voluntary movement can be detected. This interval between electrical and clinical detection of recovery is the important one in the management of the patient, and, for reasons already given, is inconstant and dependent on the chance anatomy of motor unit re-innervation. The long intervals seem to occur in muscles supplied by a nerve, e.g. the radial and facial, whose composition is predominantly motor, and may be of the order of 12–14 weeks. In an analysis of the records from nearly 500 muscles showing an electrical-clinical recovery interval, the mean interval was 29 days, the longest 121 days; 80 per cent of the observed intervals fall between 18 and 15 days (Ritchie, 1954).

Newman and Livingston (1947) found that 27 per cent of their muscle series showed voluntary trace movement before discontinuities in the I-D curve appeared; this is in reasonably good agreement with Ritchie's figure of 24 per cent, in which electrical and clinical recovery coincided. Ritchie further found that 5 per cent showed substantial clinical recovery before electrical signs appeared, and that in no case did clinical recovery occur without electrical signs becoming demonstrable within one to two weeks. This observation has little clinical importance, because, once clinical recovery has been evidenced, there is no call for the I-D curve procedure, but the facts are indicative of the spread of recordings. Moreover, in 2 per cent of cases electrical recovery was not followed by any appearance of voluntary movement, and these represent the muscles whose re-innervation ceased at the stage when sufficient motor units were available to produce a response, electrically evoked, but insufficient to produce a motor nerve controlled clinical contraction.

Wynn Parry (1954) produces records which give the average electrical-clinical recovery interval as six to eight weeks; his work was done with a low-impedance stimulator of improved accuracy over those of earlier workers, and probably represents the best results obtainable in the present state of knowledge of I-D curve recording.

As re-innervation proceeds, I-D recordings should be recorded at weekly or fortnightly intervals, and changes should be detectable if the recovery process is proceeding satisfactorily. As more muscle fibres re-innervate, the nerve component of the curve becomes more obvious; the kink in the curve becomes wider, the curve shifts towards the short-duration end of the time-scale, and the general slope (which cannot be expressed by a single index because of the discontinuity, and must be assessed by graphical plotting) becomes less steep (Wynn Parry, 1961).

During the process of degeneration, similar changes are seen, occurring in the reverse direction; but, of course, the overall time-scale is extremely variable with differences in the nature of the pathological causes. Wynn Parry (1961) says that the I-D curve shows the double curve of partial innervation after two to three days, and the typical denervated curve within fourteen days; these observations refer to complete and sudden lesions, for he further points out that, in gradual denervation such as neuritis or compression, discontinuities in the I-D curve may record small regions of denervation before any clinical manifestation of motor weakness or sensory loss.

6
Electrical Stimulation:
Accommodation Measurements

The methods considered in Chapter 5 have been concerned with the use of electrical shocks where the application was sudden and the rate of rise very high. In addition to intensity and duration of a stimulus, there is another factor that determines its effectiveness, and this is the rate of the rise of the wave-front.

If a stimulus of gradually increasing intensity is applied to excitable tissue, a very high value may be reached before excitation or 'triggering of response' takes place. Living tissue has the power of adapting or accommodating its polarised structure to a gradual strain in such a way that a shock sufficient to cause excitation if applied suddenly may be quite inadequate if the peak of the stimulus is reached over a period of time; thus, the threshold value for excitation by a gradually increasing, or progressive, stimulus may be many times higher than the threshold for a sudden stimulus. The ratio of these threshold values is a measure of the 'accommodation' of a tissue. The accommodation powers of nerve fibre are much greater than those of muscle alone, and, as Bordet (1907) pointed out, this fact can be used to distinguish innervated from denervated muscle.

Accommodation measurement as a diagnostic procedure has been little used in this country, and the concept and methods are unfamiliar, but a number of workers (Solandt, 1935, 1936; Kugelberg, 1944; Pollock *et al.*, 1944, 1945; Pollock *et al.*, 1945) have described techniques and series of case records.

There are a number of methods which, while all basically dependent on the assessment of accommodation, differ sufficiently to justify separate description. It should be noted that accommodation, while innately related to the structure of nerve and muscle and to excitability characteristics in general, requires special methods for its measurement; it cannot be deduced directly from I-D curve recordings. Keith Lucas (1907) established a quantitative relationship between rate of increase of stimulus and response, effectively showing that a 'minimal current gradient' was necessary for excitation to occur at all.

Liberson (1934), and later Kugelberg (1944), extended these observations to human nerve, and demonstrated that the minimal current gradient only applies within limits and that increase of stimulus strength beyond a certain value causes a breakdown of accommodation (*see also* Bernhard *et al.*, Skoglund, 1942).

The unit in general use for the expression of accommodation is that due to Hill (1936), who proposed a 'time constant of accommodation' referred to as lambda (λ) and defined as the reciprocal of minimum current slope. Lambda is expressed in time units, and varies between 40 and 100 msec for normal innervated human muscle; the value is affected not only by neuromuscular disorders but by metabolic changes such as occur in tetany and hypothermia (Solandt, 1936; Simpson, 1955).

GALVANIC-TETANUS RATIO
This test involves the production of sustained contraction in muscle by continuous galvanic current. This is to some extent an unphysiological procedure, but it has the advantage of simplicity in that the ordinary galvanic current can be used without modification. The rheobase is first determined, that is, the threshold excitability of the muscle to a random shock of about one second's duration. A galvanic current is then applied through the same electrodes, and is gradually increased in strength until continuous contraction takes place, when the value is recorded. The ratio, current required to produce tetanus rheobase, is of the order of five for normal muscle and less than two for denervated muscle. No attempt is made in this test to measure or standardise the rate of increase.

Provided that the sustained contraction is limited to a few seconds at most—long enough to read the meter, and no more—the procedure is reasonably well tolerated by patients, and is simple and rapid. Nevertheless, the test is hazardous for the subject. It is one of the few diagnostic measures liable to produce skin burns, because of the high and prolonged current sometimes needed to produce contraction.

PROGRESSIVE CURRENT TESTING
Accurate measurement of accommodation requires a stimulus source capable of delivering a gradually increasing shock, where the period

of rise and peak value at the threshold of excitation can be recorded. The configuration in time of the rising wave-front is of some importance. Currents that increase exponentially, logarithmically or linearly, may be used.

But wave-forms which increase other than linearly have the considerable disadvantage that the rate of rise is variable, and often indeterminate at the moment of excitation; moreover, a wave-front which rises to a measurable value and is then suddenly terminated may give rise to a 'break' excitation because of the rapid reduction to zero of the high threshold intensity level reached by the gradual stimulus. From the technical aspect, these waves are relatively simple to produce by means of resistance-capacitance circuits, and have been commonly employed; the discrepancies in reported results can often be attributed to a failure to appreciate the importance of the applied pulse shape and the impedance of the generator which supplies it.

The use of technically sophisticated stimulators capable of delivering outputs of known impedance and true isosceles-triangle configuration, variable in amplitude and in base width, will be referred to later.

It is not advisable to use a progressive-current method alone, that is to say, merely recording the threshold at which excitation occurs. If the rheobase of the particular muscle is already high, the excitation value to progressive current may be extremely so. The important index of accommodation is the ratio threshold for progressive current/threshold for sudden-shock excitation. This ratio expresses the relative elevation of threshold when the stimulus is gradual as opposed to instantaneous, and is a true measurement of accommodation.

Satisfactory commercial apparatus for this test is not available, but numerous circuits have been published (Solandt, 1935; Kugelberg, 1944; Osborne et al., 1944) which vary somewhat in their characteristic. Solandt describes a simple arrangement for producing exponentially increasing shocks of relatively short duration (fractions of a second), which are suitable for normal nerve-muscle, but ineffective for denervated muscle except at very high intensities. The other authors employ more complex and refined techniques, electronic in the case of Kugelberg and Grodins, and electro-mechanical in the instance of Pollock, for producing progressive current shocks of long duration (several seconds) with linear wave-fronts. Both

Kugelberg and Pollock have published good reviews of the history and literature of this method. Pollock *et al.* (1945*a*) have published an important paper dealing with electro-diagnosis of peripheral nerve injury by such currents, and this remains the principal source of clinical information.

The method is not a simple one for routine testing; there is some difficulty in determining the exact intensity for constant response, the muscular contraction being usually of a prolonged or tetanic nature when it occurs. The objection already made to galvanic tetanus ratio determination also applies here, in that considerable currents may have to be applied for several seconds; it frequently happens that the stimulus has to be repeated a number of times to check the observations, and care is required to avoid tissue injury.

Although little employed in this country the claims made for the accuracy of a long-duration progressive-current diagnostic test are impressive, and will be considered later. The method must be considered seriously as an important contribution to electro-diagnosis.

ALTERNATING CURRENT INTENSITY—FREQUENCY CURVES

In so far as duration of stimulus and rate of rise of its 'attack' are both factors in excitation measurement, it is to be expected on theoretical grounds that stimulation with sinusoidal alternating current of variable frequency will demonstrate a definite optimum frequency for a particular type of tissue. This optimum occurs when the frequency of alternation is such that the combination of rate of rise and half-wave duration balance out, so to speak, in effectiveness. At frequencies below the optimum, the rate of rise will be slow; at higher frequencies the duration of each half-cycle will be short. From the aspect of effective stimulation the two oppose each other.

The application of variable-frequency a.c. to muscle and nerve and the measurement of the intensity required at each frequency, reveals a frequency-intensity relationship which shows a definite optimal frequency. Currents of small intensity are more effective at this frequency than above or below it (Hill *et al.*, 1936; Osborne *et al.*, 1944; Grodins *et al.*, 1944). As the optimal frequency for minimum-intensity excitation is of the order of 60 c/s for normal, and 2 c/s for denervated human muscle, the diagnostic possibilities of the method are evident. Three factors have retarded the development of the method except in small-scale experiments. It is difficult and costly to procure an a.c. generator capable of delivering adequate power at the low frequencies needed for denervated muscle (0·5 to 5 c/s). The method involves continuous passage of current through tissues and the risk of burning is a real one at high intensities, for although excitation depends on frequency, tissue heating does not. Third, the optimal frequency depends to some extent on the index of response, powerful contraction of denervated muscle requiring a higher frequency than perceptible response of the same muscles (Grodins et al., 1944). It is doubtful if this latter observation represents a serious objection in careful diagnostic work, where the response is always small, but its bearing on the optimal frequency for therapeutic stimulation is most important. There are other minor technical difficulties, and the number of observations made is insufficient to justify conclusions.

Normal muscle, when tested by variable frequency sinusoidal alternating current, shows a response to 50 to 60 c/s which can be elicited at lower intensity than for any other frequency, higher or lower. It is noteworthy in this connection that 50 c/s being the usual power-line frequency in this country it is as effective and dangerous a current for causing accidental electrocution as could well be selected.

The optimum frequency point on an intensity-frequency curve is not sharp, and the threshold in general varies only about 20 per cent between 20 and 100 c/s. The test is not an easy one to apply. Patients are intolerant of continuous a.c. stimulation, and the risk of tissue damage cannot be ignored. If the current is gradually increased (at any frequency) from zero to threshold, tetanus develops so gradually that it is most difficult to assess a standard degree of contraction without elaborate mechanical aids. On the other hand, if the current is applied suddenly random effects will arise because of the exact phase at which the current is applied to the tissue; the current may be zero, or peak in either direction, or much more commonly, some intermediate value.

It appears from experiment that without considerable development, either in the way of recording muscular tension, or in respect of electronic 'keying' of the sinusoidal burst so that it commences at zero current, the method has practical difficulties; it has not been used extensively in this country. Liberson (1961) after an extensive review of principles and methods of accommodation measurement, concludes that strength-frequency determinations have not been developed to a stage satisfactory for clinical use.

CLINICAL FINDINGS

In general, no substantial series has been published to enable assessment to be considered statistically as can be done with intensity-duration curves. Most of the published work referred to contains case records, and the results obtained by different authorities are in good agreement, and may be summarised as follows:

A galvanic-tetanus ratio approaching unity is characteristic of full denervation, the muscle behaving as a contractile substance bereft of powers of accommodation. As a rheobase shock of the order of one second duration is required initially, and very little increase will produce indefinite tetanic persistence of contraction, the procedure requires care in the discernment of the minimum degree of response. It is not easy to distinguish the protracted sluggish twitch of denervated muscle from the tetanic state, as both develop slowly and locally under the electrode.

Progressive-current testing confirms the galvanic-tetanus ratio in a more quantitative manner, and in the denervated state the ratio progressive-current intensity/rheobase (for currents of several seconds' duration) approaches unity. The authorities on this method believe that careful and experienced determination of the galvanic tetanus ratio is as good a practical diagnostic measure as the more elaborate progressive-current testing, particularly as no specialised apparatus is needed.

Denervated muscle responds to the smallest threshold intensity of alternating current when the frequency is in the range of 0·5 to 2 c/s.

Pollock et al. (1945) describe the results of the examination of over fifty cases of peripheral nerve injury. When electrical signs of recovery appeared, the later course of events confirmed their validity in all but seven cases, in five of which information was not forthcoming. Only two cases presented equivocal findings. In all the cases that were diagnosed electrically as denervated the observation was confirmed by other means. Pollock and his co-workers believe that a very high accommodation ratio or a very high galvanic threshold appearing from a muscle assessed as denervated (low ratio: low threshold) are indicative of regeneration, and their results show this to be a valuable practical observation. They do not give a detailed account of the electrical-clinical recovery interval, except to comment that the longest observed interval was 150 days.

In a later paper (Pollock et al., 1945b), they express the opinion

7

that determination of galvanic-tetanus ratio is probably diagnostically as effective, and practically simpler.

Newman and Livingston (1947) comparing simultaneous records of I-D curves, note that I-D curve discontinuities appeared in 54 per cent of their cases, and that the electrical-clinical recovery interval averaged ninety-seven days: 48 per cent of the same cases showed a rise of galvanic-tetanus ratio, averaging 109 days before clinical motor recovery. Taking the two tests together, a reliable prognosis was given in 73 per cent of cases.

TRIANGULAR PULSE INTENSITY-DURATION RECORDING

Within the last few years, improvements in electronic techniques have made it possible to produce, at least for research purposes, stimulators which deliver triangular pulses of variable duration and intensity. The recordings from these detect changes in the threshold and accommodation time constant of affected muscle, changes which are not revealed by I-D curves plotted with rectangular 'sudden shock' waveforms.

The triangular wave-form is capable of selective stimulation of denervated muscle, and the method has important uses in connection with therapeutic stimulation (Thom, 1953); the diagnostic possibilities have been recently examined in a preliminary paper by Stephens (in press). His stimulator of sophisticated design, delivering true triangular pulses variable in duration from 0·1 msec to 1 sec, and of intensities variable from 0 to 100 mA, had calibration accuracies on all scales of better than one per cent of full scale. It is of interest to note that Stephens adopted the high-impedance current-calibrated output (2–5 MΩ) in this instrument, because the discomfort problem does not arise with pulses of sloping wave-front; the sensory elements in the skin and tissues accommodate, and are not readily depolarized by triangular pulses.

The basis of the method is to record intensity-duration curves with pulses of *triangular* configuration, and such curves show a sharply defined optimal duration/minimum intensity. At longer durations of triangular pulse the current increases too slowly and tissues accommodate; at shorter durations the quantity of electricity/pulse is inadequate for stimulation.

Using the data supplied by Desmedt (1950), obtained from careful experimental study on rabbit muscle during the course of degeneration and regeneration, Stephens has computed response curves for triangular pulse stimulation of nerve, muscle, and denervated muscle.

Preliminary clinical observation demonstrates good agreement between observed and predicted curves, and the technique facilitates detection of early signs of denervation and progression of degenerative changes; these are, in general, not well revealed by conventional methods.

While the authors regard it as important to refer to this development as one which has valuable clinical potentialities, it cannot yet, without further clinical trial, be regarded as of established value. Nevertheless, it is worthwhile to appreciate that despite the long history and extensive practice of orthodox electro-diagnostic stimulation, advances may yet be expected.

7
Nerve Trauma and Compression Syndromes

Nerve trauma may take the form of sudden contusion or section of a peripheral nerve as the result of acute injury or of a localised chronic neuropathy due to pressure on a nerve by neighbouring tissues, where it lies in a confined space (Kopell and Thompson, 1963). The first type of injury, although it occurs not uncommonly in civilian life, received intensive study during the Second World War. The frequency of the pressure neuropathies has become evident comparatively recently, and their analysis has been greatly assisted by electrophysiological techniques.

Peripheral nerve trauma presents, in the first instance, as a defect in one or all of the three functional components of a mixed nerve, motor, sensory, or autonomic. While the initial diagnosis is made on clinical assessment of these functions, and the site of the lesion, where not immediately obvious, is determined by considerations of anatomical innervation of skin and muscle, many aspects of nerve injury call for more precise examination. In acute peripheral nerve injuries, electrical methods of study are particularly valuable in the early stages in assessing the severity of the nerve damage and, in the later stages, in determining the prognosis and in predicting recovery in advance of clinical assessment. In the pressure neuropathies, the value of electrophysiological methods is largely in confirming the diagnosis where this is doubtful, and in giving precise localisation to the site of the nerve lesion. In acute nerve injury, the most useful methods of study have been the evaluation of denervation by motor point stimulation using the strength-duration curve technique and concentric electrode electromyography. In the study of the pressure neuropathies, nerve conduction measurement has provided particularly useful information.

NATURE AND EFFECTS OF NERVE INJURY, COURSE, AND PROGNOSIS

Injuries to peripheral nerve may be classified according to whether the damage causes nothing more than a temporary conduction block,

84

or whether it is severe enough to cause local destruction of the axon at the site of injury, with consequent Wallerian degeneration. The first type of injury has been called neurapraxia. The second is known as axonotmesis if local destruction of the axon occurs but the connective tissue of the nerve is intact, or neurotmesis where the whole thickness of the nerve is divided (Seddon, 1943). These distinctions are of clinical as well as pathological significance. In neurapraxia, recovery may be rapid as the local effects of injury subside. Following axonotmesis and neurotmesis, recovery can only take place by the process of regeneration by which the axon slowly grows down the endoneurium at a rate approaching 3·0 mm/day. Regeneration following axonotmesis may be uncomplicated and eventually complete. Following neurotmesis, recovery may be further delayed because it does not begin until a neuroma has formed at the site of the lesion. It may be complicated, because after nerve section some axons may regrow along the distal segments which originally belonged to other axons, and recovery is frequently incomplete. In a damaged peripheral nerve, neurapraxia and axonotmesis may coexist, giving rise to partial denervation.

Neurapraxia occurs comparatively infrequently as the result of acute trauma in civilian life, but is a common sequel to mild continued pressure and it is a feature of many of the pressure or entrapment neuropathies. Relatively little information is available from clinical studies regarding the pathological changes which affect the nerve, but experimental work on animals has shown that there may be swelling and local oedema of the nerve together with thinning and local dissolution of the myelin (Denny-Brown and Brenner, 1944). It may be that it is this localised loss of myelin that accounts for the local impairment of conduction velocity, which is frequently a feature of entrapment neuropathies.

Following section of a nerve, the distal segment remains excitable for a period of several days. If the excitability of a muscle is measured after complete nerve section by determining the magnitude of stimuli which will excite it and recording the strength-duration curves, a change in excitability to short duration (100 μsec) pulses may be detected as early as the third day, and a curve consistent with denervation is obtained at about the fifth or sixth day. If the nerve is stimulated remote from the muscle, it is possible to evoke a visible twitch of the muscle for three to four days after nerve section. If the evoked potentials are recorded from the muscle, these may still be recorded for up to about seven days after nerve section. The conduction velocity along the degenerating segment of nerve shows little if any reduction (Landau, 1953; Gilliatt and Taylor, 1959).

It is evident that the strength-duration curve gives particularly early evidence of denervation after a peripheral nerve lesion, but conduction velocity measurement must be interpreted with caution at this stage, since evoked potentials of normal or nearly normal latency may be obtained for several days after a complete nerve lesion. At this time, the attenuated character of the evoked potential is of more value than its latency. Electromyography with concentric electrodes is, at this stage, of relatively limited value. A failure to obtain action potentials on attempted contraction may be misleading, since the production of a voluntary contraction depends on the co-operation of the patient. Objective evidence of denervation in the form of fibrillation and positive sharp waves may occur as early as five days after nerve injury, but it is more frequently delayed, not appearing for two to three weeks.

During regeneration of a nerve, both the strength duration curve and the exploration of a muscle with a concentric electrode may give advance information of recovery an appreciable period before there is any visible sign of voluntary contraction. The first evidence of re-innervation provided by the strength duration curve is the appearance of a kink or discontinuity in a curve which previously was of denervated type. A discontinuity in the curve may be demonstrated two to four months before there is clinical evidence of recovery. The first electromyographic sign of re-innervation is the appearance of brief low amplitude potentials (less than 3 msec and 300 μV), which may anticipate clinical recovery by two to four months. About three weeks later, complex, frequently polyphasic, potentials of longer duration make their appearance. These potentials are most easily recorded from the vicinity of the motor point, and, in later stages, are succeeded by polyphasic potentials of very much greater amplitude and duration (12 to 16 msec and 1 to 2 mV). As more segments of the muscle undergo re-innervation, the number of motor units recruited during voluntary contraction increases until, if recovery is complete or nearly complete, an interference pattern will be evident on maximal effort (Wynn Parry, 1953).

Conduction velocity studies are unhelpful during the early stages of regeneration, because no evoked potentials can be recorded until re-innervation of the muscle has commenced. For many months after clinical recovery has been apparent, conduction velocity shows marked slowing (Hodes *et al.*, 1948). Where the nerve injury has involved axonotmesis without physical separation of the proximal and distal segments, conduction velocity may eventually return to normal (Sanders and Whitteridge, 1946), but following nerve section and suture some degree of slowing of conduction velocity is likely to be permanent (Berry *et al.*, 1944).

LESIONS OF THE BRACHIAL PLEXUS

Injuries to the brachial plexus may occur as the result of birth injury, and are usually due to traction affecting either the upper or the lower part of the plexus. The commoner variety is generally due to downward traction on the arm, which may occur in a breech presentation, and the part of the plexus affected is that derived from the fifth and sixth cervical roots. It is known as Erb's paralysis. A less common injury may result from downward traction on the arm during delivery of the trunk in a vertex presentation. In this the lower plexus derived from C.8 and T.1 roots is involved, and the condition is known as Klumpke's paralysis. In adult life, injuries, especially if there is severe and sudden traction on the shoulder, may lead either to an upper or a lower plexus lesion, and sometimes the whole plexus is affected. In severe cases, the cervical roots may be avulsed from the cord. In bronchogenic carcinoma, the brachial plexus may be invaded by tumour (Pancoast's tumour) and deep X-ray therapy may occasionally result in post radiation fibrosis affecting the plexus. A common local lesion of the brachial plexus is the cervical rib syndrome where the medial cord of the brachial plexus, sometimes together with the subclavian artery may be compressed between a rib or fibrous band, arising from the C.7 transverse process, and the scalenus muscle. The condition is aggravated by age and by weakness of the shoulder girdle muscles, which allows the shoulders to sag, and the muscles affected are those supplied by C.8 and T.1. There are frequently paraesthesiae and some sensory loss.

The analysis of brachial plexus lesions depends principally on careful clinical testing of muscle power, and the distribution of sensory loss. Electromyography and strength duration curves can give useful additional information by showing the distribution of partial denervation. In partial lesions, the amount of motor unit activity on voluntary contraction is helpful in assessing the severity of the lesion and estimating the prognosis. Serial examinations are useful in that changes in the strength-duration curves, and the return of motor unit activity, may give advance information regarding recovery.

Motor conduction velocity is frequently unhelpful in brachial plexus lesions, since motor conduction velocity may be normal unless the lesion is a total one, in which case no evoked potentials can be recorded. Conduction latencies in the proximal parts of the plexus can be measured by stimulating the trunks of the plexus at Erb's point, in the angle between the posterior border of sterno-mastoid and the clavicle at the level of the sixth cervical vertebra. Evoked potentials may be recorded from the muscles of the shoulder and the proximal part of the upper limb. Using this technique, little abnormality in latency may be found in brachial plexus injuries in contrast to what is found in peripheral neuropathy (Gassel, 1964). On the other hand, sensory nerve action potentials may be lost in brachial plexus injuries. In the cervical rib syndrome, the sensory potential from the fifth finger may be lost, whereas in lesions of the whole plexus it may not be possible to evoke sensory potentials by stimulation of any fingers on the affected side (Gilliatt, 1961). Where the roots are avulsed from the cord in severe brachial plexus injuries, the first sensory neurone may be preserved and sensory action potentials may be recorded from both median and ulnar nerves in spite of complete anaesthesia (Bonney and Gilliatt, 1958).

PRESSURE AND ENTRAPMENT NEUROPATHIES

Few major peripheral nerves are not subject to compression or recurrent trauma at vulnerable points along their course (Fig. 7.1). Mononeuropathies due to nerve entrapment may give rise to symptoms which initially cause only minor distress, and for which the diagnosis may be obscure if careful attention is not given to the anatomical localisation of the symptoms, in terms of the distribution of a single peripheral nerve or branch of a nerve. Electromyography by showing signs of partial denervation in muscles supplied by a particular nerve may provide confirmatory evidence, but the most valuable method of investigating the possibility of local peripheral nerve pathology is by measurement of nerve conduction velocity. This is so because, in many instances, the nerve damage amounts to no more than a simple conduction block without Wallerian degeneration or signs of denervation. Moreover, the delay in nerve

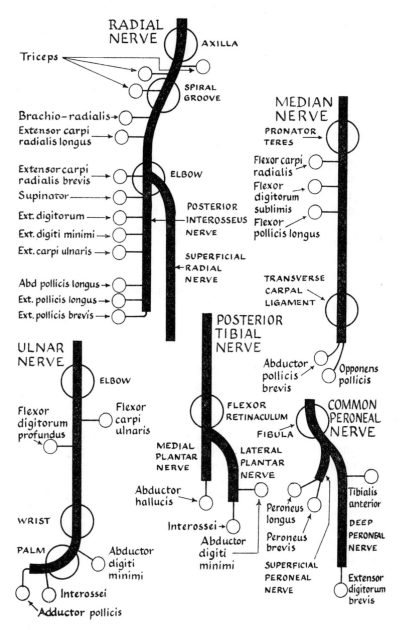

FIGURE 7.1 Diagram to illustrate the common sites where nerve compression or injury may occur in five peripheral nerves which are readily accessible to nerve conduction measurement. The large circles indicate the common sites for nerve injury.

conduction may sometimes be localised to a small segment of nerve near the site of compression, with relatively normal conduction velocity proximal and distal to the lesion. Demonstration of a local conduction block in this way may not only assist in establishing the diagnosis but also provide guidance regarding possible surgical treatment. Following surgical decompression of a peripheral nerve, serial conduction velocity measurements are of value in the assessment of progress because, in many instances after successful decompression, conduction velocity gradually reverts to normal (Goodman and Gilliatt, 1961).

While many entrapment neuropathies have a single mechanical cause, there are many generalised disorders which may affect peripheral nerves and may render them particularly vulnerable to trauma (Mulder et al., 1960). It is therefore important, whenever nerve conduction studies are carried out on suspected cases of compression neuropathy, to study nerves other than those which appear to be clinically affected.

THE MEDIAN NERVE

The median nerve is derived from the lateral and medial cords of the brachial plexus and receives fibres from C.6, 7, 8, and T.1 roots. It is a mixed nerve supplying muscles in the forearm and hand, and the skin over the palmar aspect of the thumb, index, and middle fingers, and the lateral aspect of the ring finger, and it also contains many autonomic vasomotor fibres. It enters the forearm by passing between the ulnar and humeral heads of pronator teres, and then gives off the anterior interosseus branch. In the forearm it supplies pronator teres, flexor carpi radialis, palmaris longus, and flexor digitorum sublimis. The anterior interosseus branch supplies flexor pollicis longus, the lateral half of flexor digitorum profundus, and pronator quadratus. The median nerve enters the hand by passing through the carpal tunnel under the transverse carpal ligament, and supplies abductor pollicis brevis, flexor pollicis brevis, and opponens pollicis in the thenar eminence, and also the first and second lumbricals.

The most important site of injury to the median nerve is at the wrist as it passes through the carpal tunnel, but it may also be injured at the elbow where it passes between the two heads of pronator teres. Injury to the median nerve at the wrist may follow a Colles fracture, and common conditions which may be associated with the carpal tunnel syndrome are rheumatoid arthritis, tenosynovitis, pregnancy, and myxoedema. Clinically, the salient features are painful paraesthesiae in the median nerve distribution and often associated with vasomotor disturbance (acroparaesthesiae), frequently awakening the patient at night. There may be sensory impairment in the hand and wasting of the thenar eminence, and weakness of abduction and opposition of the thumb.

The carpal tunnel syndrome was the earliest of the pressure neuropathies to be studied by nerve conduction velocity measurement (Simpson, 1956). Motor conduction is readily measured by stimulating the median nerve at the wrist and recording evoked potentials from the thenar muscles, either with a concentric electrode or with surface electrodes. The normal latency at the wrist is 2 to 4 msec, and a latency of greater than 4·5 msec, or one that is significantly greater than that of the contralateral side, is evidence that the nerve may be compressed in the carpal tunnel. If the median nerve is stimulated in the forearm or in the cubital fossa, subtraction of the distal from the proximal latent period makes it possible to calculate the conduction velocity from elbow to wrist. The diagnosis of carpal tunnel syndrome is strengthened if prolonged latency at the wrist can be shown to be associated with normal conduction velocity from elbow to wrist. However, in a considerable number of cases there is also slowing of nerve conduction proximal to the carpal tunnel (Thomas, 1960). Experimental work has shown that after nerve crush, slowing of nerve conduction may take place in the proximal part of the nerve (Cragg and Thomas, 1964). While slowing of nerve conduction in the proximal part of the median nerve is thus compatible with a carpal tunnel syndrome, its presence is an indication for more detailed examination. It may, for example, mean that the carpal tunnel syndrome is part of a more widespread neuropathy, due perhaps to diabetes or polyarteritis nodosa (Fig. 7.2). It can also mean that the pressure palsy may arise at a more proximal site, such as the pronator teres muscle.

Although the majority of established cases of carpal tunnel syndrome show a prolonged latency at the wrist, the latency is normal in a considerable number of cases. In the presence of normal latency, however, the character of the evoked potential may be abnormal, with increase in both the total duration and the number of phases on account of temporal dispersion of the summated action potential. Repetitive firing, that is a series of evoked potentials occurring after a single stimulus, occurs in a proportion of cases (Simpson, 1956). The significance of repetitive firing is that it indicates altered excitability in a damaged segment of nerve. In normal subjects, it may occur during or following ischaemia and in hypocalcaemia (Kugelberg, 1946). Cases which show normal or only slightly impaired motor latency may show abnormalities in the sensory evoked potential, following stimulation of the fingers with ring electrodes (Gilliatt and Sears, 1958). The nerve action potential at the wrist may be of reduced amplitude or absent. The latency may also be prolonged but, if the

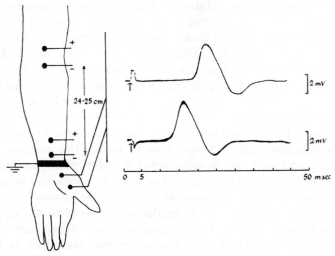

FIGURE 7.2 Motor conduction measurement in the median nerve of a diabetic patient with the carpal tunnel syndrome. The latency of 10·0 msec between the stimulus at the wrist and the evoked potential is greatly prolonged. Since the latency after stimulation at the elbow is 16·0 msec and the distance between the stimulating cathodes 24·25 cm the conduction velocity elbow to wrist is 40·4 m/s.

potential is markedly delayed, it may not be possible to record it on account of the marked temporal dispersion of its components which occurs. Electromyographic examination of the wasted muscles with a concentric electrode, by showing signs of partial denervation confined to muscles supplied by the median nerve, may provide confirmatory evidence of the diagnosis (Marinacci, 1964).

THE ULNAR NERVE

The ulnar nerve is a continuation of the medial cord of the brachial plexus, and contains fibres derived from C.8 and T.1 roots. In the upper arm, it passes between the biceps and triceps muscles in close relation to the brachial artery and median nerve, and it passes through a groove behind the medial epicondyle of the humerus to reach the forearm. In the forearm, it supplies the flexor carpi ulnaris and the medial half of flexor digitorum profundus. After entering the hand it divides into a superficial and a deep branch. The superficial branch supplies the skin over the hypothenar eminence, and the palmar surface of the fifth finger, and the medial aspect of the ring finger. The deep branch has no sensory supply, and near its origin gives off branches to supply the hypothenar muscles. After curving laterally round the hook of the hamate it supplies the interossei, and third and fourth lumbricals, and the adductor pollicis.

The commonest site for an ulnar nerve lesion is at the elbow, where it lies in a groove behind the medial epicondyle of the humerus. Injury to the ulnar nerve in this situation occurs readily from external trauma, and gradual damage may occur if the nerve is stretched against the ulnar groove, as it may be if there is a significant degree of valgus deformity as may result from fractures near the elbow. Occupation pressure on the nerve may be aggravated by ostero-arthritis at the elbow joint. The most prominent symptoms of an ulnar neuropathy are weakness and wasting of the intrinsic muscles of the hand, often particularly marked in the first dorsal interosseus muscle. There may be impairment of sensation over the fifth finger and the medial aspect of the fourth finger.

In lesions of the ulnar nerve, at the elbow, there may be localised slowing of nerve conduction over the affected segment of the ulnar nerve, with relatively normal conduction velocity in the proximal and distal segments of the nerve (Simpson, 1956). More frequently, the proximal portion of the nerve shows relatively normal conduction velocity, but there is some degree of slowing in the whole nerve distal to the elbow (Gilliatt and Thomas, 1960). The ulnar nerve is relatively accessible to electrical stimulation from the axilla to the wrist, and the muscles of the hand can be readily activated by stimuli at different situations along its course. Nerve action potentials can also be recorded at various points, following stimulation of the fingers with ring electrodes or of the ulnar nerve itself at the wrist or elbow. In ulnar nerve lesions at the elbow, nerve action potentials evoked by stimulating at the fingers or wrist may be unobtainable, but may sometimes be recorded in the axilla if the nerve is stimulated immediately above the elbow (Gilliatt and Thomas, 1960).

The ulnar nerve may be damaged as it enters the hand, and in this clinical situation the signs are similar to those of an ulnar nerve lesion at the elbow, with weakness of the intrinsic muscles and sensory loss. Damage to the deep branch (Fig. 7.3) may occur through external trauma, sometimes resulting from occupational pressure on the palm or, not uncommonly, through pressure on the hand by a benign swelling such as a ganglion. Damage generally occurs distal to the origin of the branches supplying the hyopthenar muscles, and gives rise to weakness and wasting of the intrinsic muscles of the

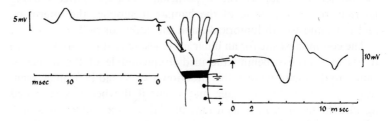

FIGURE 7.3 Neuropathy affecting the deep branch of the ulnar nerve. The latency from the wrist to abductor digiti minimi is less than 4·0 msec, whereas to the first dorsal interosseus it is greater than 9·0 msec.

hand, excepting those of the hypothenar eminence and those supplied by the median nerve, and with no loss of sensation. If the ulnar nerve is stimulated at the wrist there may be a normal latency from the wrist to the abductor digiti minimi, but an abnormally prolonged latency from the wrist to the first dorsal interosseus muscle (Simpson, 1956; Ebeling et al., 1960).

THE RADIAL NERVE

The radial nerve arises in the axilla as a continuation of the posterior cord of the brachial plexus, and receives fibres from C.5, 6, 7, 8, and T.1. In the upper arm it winds round the humerus in the spiral groove to pass from the medial to the lateral side of the arm. Before it enters the groove it gives off branches to supply the triceps and anconeous muscles. After leaving the spiral groove, it enters the forearm in front of the lateral epicondyle of the humerus between brachialis and brachioradialis, which it supplies along with extensor carpi radialis longus. In this situation, it gives off the posterior interosseus nerve of the forearm, a purely motor nerve which supplies supinator, anconeus, extensor digitorum, extensor digiti minimi, extensor carpi ulnaris, the abductor, and the long extensor of the thumb. The main branch of the radial nerve becomes superficial in the distal third of the forearm, and supplies the dorsum of the wrist and the lateral side of the dorsum of the hand.

The radial nerve may be injured in the axilla, for example, by pressure from a crutch, in which case the triceps may be paralysed. Probably the most vulnerable part of the nerve is that part which lies in the spiral groove, which may be injured by local pressure as in a 'Saturday night palsy' or by fracture of the humerus. Lower down it may be injured by a fracture of the head of the radius. The posterior interosseus nerve may be injured as it passes through the supinator muscle, and this may cause motor weakness without sensory loss.

Electrical stimulation of the radial nerve is less readily accomplished than is the case with the median and ulnar nerves, and electromyographic exploration of muscles supplied by the radial nerve, for signs of denervation, is of particular value in studying possible lesions of the radial nerve. Motor conduction velocity can be measured by stimulating the trunks of the brachial plexus in the posterior triangle of the neck (Erb's Point), and stimulating the radial nerve distally either in the spiral groove or where the nerve becomes superficial at the lateral aspect of the humerus. Evoked potentials may be recorded if concentric electrodes are placed in anconeus, brachioradialis, and the extensor digitorum muscles (Gassel and Diamantopoulos, 1964).

A useful approach to conduction velocity measurement has been to stimulate the superficial sensory branch of the radial nerve where it becomes superficial in the forearm, so as to record antidromic sensory potentials from the distal part of the nerve at the base of the thumb. This method may show abnormalities in the radial nerve arising from lesions at, or above, the elbow, but it gives no information in lesions affecting the posterior interosseus nerve (Downie and Scott, 1967).

THE FEMORAL NERVE

The fermoral nerve is derived from the second, third, and fourth segments of the lumbar plexus, and after passing through the psoas muscle it enters the thigh under the inguinal ligament. It supplies pectineus, sartorius, and quadriceps femoris, and the skin over the front of the thigh through the medial and intermediate nerves of the thigh. Lesions of the femoral nerve may be difficult to distinguish from lesions of the lumbar plexus. The nerve may be involved by retroperitoneal neoplasm, or injured by inflammation or haemorrhage in the psoas muscle. A mononeuritis affecting the femoral nerve may occur particularly in diabetes. In addition to wasting and weakness of the quadriceps, a femoral neuropathy may be associated with pain and sensory loss over the anterior aspect of the thigh. Disuse atrophy of the quadriceps is a frequent accompaniment of prolonged immobilisation.

Electromyography of the quadriceps is of value in distinguishing weakness due to neuropathy from myopathy affecting the quadriceps and from disuse atrophy (Thage, 1965). Measurement of conduction velocity along the femoral nerve is of value in identifying an isolated femoral neuropathy, or one which is part of a more widespread neuropathy. Femoral nerve conduction velocity can be measured by stimulating the femoral nerve at the inguinal ligament, and recording evoked potentials at successively distal sites along the rectus femoris muscle. This procedure is possible because the rectus femoris is a bipennate muscle originating from a thin central tendon, so that the end plate zone forms a largely vertical band along the muscle (Gassel, 1963; Chopra and Hurwitz, 1968). In this nerve Gassel (1963) has recorded a normal mean conduction velocity of 70 m/sec ±7·8 per cent.

THE COMMON PERONEAL NERVE
The common peroneal (lateral popliteal) nerve is derived from L.4, L.5, S.1 and 2 roots of the lumbo-sacral plexus, and arises at the bifurcation of the sciatic nerve in the popliteal fossa. It enters the leg by winding round the lateral aspect of the head of the fibula, and passing through an opening in the origin of peroneus longus. In this situation, the nerve is exposed to trauma and this is one of the commonest sites of pressure neuropathy in the body. As it enters the leg it divides into three terminal divisions, the superficial peroneal (musculo-cutaneous), the deep peroneal (anterior tibial), and the recurrent peroneal nerves. The superior peroneal nerve supplies peroneus longus and brevis. The deep peroneal supplies tibialis anterior, extensor digitorum longus, extensor hallucis longus, peroneus tertius, and extensor digitorum brevis. The superficial and deep peroneal nerves supply sensation to the skin over the dorsum of the foot, and the lateral surface of the distal part of the leg.

The most common cause of injury to the common peroneal

nerve is damage caused by compression of the nerve between the head of the fibula and the opposite knee when the legs are crossed. It is particularly liable to occur in thin persons who have lost weight. At the head of the fibula the nerve lies so superficially that it may frequently be exposed to direct trauma, and as is the case with other mononeuropathies, a neuropathy may occur in the presence of a systemic disorder which renders the nerve particularly vulnerable. A tightly applied plaster may compress the nerve against the head of the fibula. The most prominent clinical effect is generally weakness of dorsiflexion of the ankle, which may progress to complete foot-drop, and there may be sensory loss over the dorsum of the foot.

Electromyography with a concentric electrode inserted into the tibialis anterior may reveal signs of partial denervation in severe lesions. Motor nerve conduction studies may assist in distinguishing common peroneal lesions from symptoms due to root compression or a lesion of the lumbo-sacral plexus. Conduction velocity can readily be measured by stimulating the nerve at the head of the fibula and above the ankle, and recording evoked potentials, which can be done easily with surface electrodes, from extensor digitorum brevis. Nerve action potentials can also be recorded from the common peroneal nerve at the head of the fibula, but it is difficult to do this with surface electrodes and it is more satisfactory to use subcutaneous needles close to the nerve. The potentials are most easily evoked by stimulation of the nerve at the dorsum of the ankle, so that the potential obtained is a mixed sensory and antidromic motor action potential. With this technique nerve potentials may be of diminished amplitude, or absent in common peroneal nerve lesions and in peripheral neuropathy, in contrast to conditions such as severe motor neurone disease where normal or nearly normal potentials may be obtained even when no excitable motor fibres can be identified (Gilliatt *et al.*, 1961).

THE POSTERIOR TIBIAL NERVE

The posterior tibial nerve is the continuation of the medial popliteal nerve and starts at the lower border of popliteus. It is derived from L.4, 5, and S.1, 2, and 3 segments, and supplies tibialis posterior, flexor digitorum longus, and flexor hallucis longus. It passes into the foot between the medial malleolus and the flexor retinaculum, and divides into the medial and lateral plantar nerves, which are homologous with the median and ulnar nerves in the hand.

8

An entrapment neuropathy can affect the posterior tibial nerve where it passes in relation to the medial malleolus, and is known as the tarsal tunnel syndrome. It may develop without any history of trauma and is sometimes associated with tenosynovitis within the tarsal tunnel, and venous engorgement of the posterior tibial veins which may be related to proximal venous obstruction or stasis. The predominant symptom is pain affecting the toes and sole of the foot, and sometimes the calcaneum, and there may be sensory impairment.

Conduction velocity in the posterior tibial nerve may be studied by recording evoked potentials from the abductor hallucis. If the posterior tibial nerve is stimulated at or above the malleolus, a distal latency may be recorded and conduction velocity in the proximal part of the nerve can be calculated, if the medial popliteal nerve is stimulated in the popliteal fossa.

8
The Spinal Muscular Atrophies and Peripheral Neuropathy

In the assessment of muscular weakness, electromyography is of value in differentiating weakness due to muscle disease from weakness due to disorders of the nervous system. In neurogenic weakness the changes are most specific in disease affecting the lower motor neurone, and it is frequently possible both to establish the existence of a lower motor neurone lesion, and to distinguish between a process primarily affecting the anterior horn cells in the spinal cord and one affecting the spinal roots or the peripheral nerves. In making such a distinction, information is most readily obtained if electromyographic studies are carried out in association with nerve conduction velocity measurement.

In the case of spastic weakness due to disease affecting the upper motor neurone the findings on electromyography are less specific. On voluntary contraction of an affected muscle there may be a reduction in motor unit activity, suggesting a neurogenic disorder, and on passive stretch of the muscle, action potentials may be evoked indicating some augmentation of the stretch reflex. The electrophysiological analysis of spasticity, however, requires more complex methods. One method that has been extensively studied is the determination of the recovery cycle of the H reflex, when this is evoked by paired stimuli occurring at predetermined intervals. While this method has provided much information which is of theoretical interest, its clinical value remains to be assessed.

In this chapter various types of spinal muscular atrophy will first be considered. In later sections peripheral neuropathy will be discussed.

The Spinal Muscular Atrophies
This includes acute virus infections by a neurotropic virus such as poliomyelitis, in which the principal damage may affect the anterior horns of the grey matter of the spinal cord, progressive system

degenerations such as motor neurone disease, and hereditary conditions such as peroneal muscular atrophy, infantile spinal muscular atrophy, or Werdnig Hoffmann disease, and the Kugelberg Welander syndrome. Localised destruction of anterior horn cells may occur in spinal cord compression, vascular lesions of the cord, and intramedullary anomalies such as syringomyelia.

Certain electromyographic findings are common to these disorders. First, signs of denervation may be present in the form of excessive insertion activity, fibrillation potentials, positive sharp waves, and reduced motor unit recruitment on voluntary contraction. The strength duration curve may show a denervation pattern or present discontinuities. On the whole, however, fibrillation tends to be a less constant finding in anterior horn cell disease than in other forms of denervation atrophy. Second, in addition to single fibre activity at rest, large motor unit action potentials are frequently seen occurring, apparently spontaneously, and these may be associated with visible involuntary muscle twitches or fasciculations. On voluntary contraction the motor unit action potentials are frequently enlarged, showing an increase both in duration and in amplitude (see Chapter 2, Plate 7A). During a maximal contraction, it is characteristic to recognise these 'giant units' occurring as discrete entities in the absence of any interference pattern. If the muscle is explored with more than one electrode, motor unit action potentials may be recorded synchronously in different parts of the muscle (Buchthal and Clemmeson, 1943).

The large motor unit action potentials that are seen are associated with a corresponding increase in size of the motor units themselves, which in anterior horn cell disease comes about through the surviving axons giving off collateral sprouts, which grow out to re-innervate denervated muscle fibres (Wohlfart, 1958; Coërs and Woolf, 1959). It is possible that this enlargement of the motor units may account, at least in some measure, for synchronisation (see Chapter 3), since apparent synchronisation could result from two electrodes recording simultaneous potentials from the same abnormally large motor unit (Denny-Brown, 1949). However, it is doubtful if the territory filled by the enlarged units is adequate to account for all cases of synchronisation, and another possible explanation is that the Renshaw inhibitory loop has the effect of bringing about synchronisation, when the size of the motor neurone pool is markedly reduced as a result of anterior horn cell disease (Simpson, 1966).

POLIOMYELITIS

It is generally possible to record electrophysiological abnormalities in the affected muscles of patients with poliomyelitis during the first month after the onset of weakness. Probably the earliest abnormality to appear is in the strength-duration curve, which may show evidence of partial denervation as early as the tenth day and complete denervation by the fourteenth day (Rushworth, 1963). Fibrillation potentials may also appear during the first month after the development of symptoms, and may be associated with an excess of insertion activity and positive sharp waves. In some muscles, denervation may be complete and, in these, fibrillation can be recorded throughout the entire substance of the muscle, and on attempted voluntary contraction no motor unit action potentials will be seen. More frequently denervation is incomplete; in this event, while fibrillation may be present during relaxation, there will be partial recruitment of motor unit action potentials during attempted voluntary contraction. In partially denervated muscles, fasciculation potentials which are sometimes abnormally large and polyphasic may be seen.

At an early stage after the development of weakness, measurement of the action potential size in patients with poliomyelitis shows an increase both in mean amplitude and mean duration (Pinelli and Buchthal, 1951) This is most prominent in severely affected muscles and in the later stages of the disease. In patients examined a long interval after the development of symptoms, severely affected muscles are seen to contain an excess of large units, which may reach an amplitude of the order of 10 mV, and which are still recognisable as separate discrete potentials even on maximal effort. At quite an early stage of the disease, recording from electrodes at different sites in the muscle may show action potentials which appear to occur synchronously.

During a sustained voluntary contraction, there is a tendency for the large polyphasic units to decrease in amplitude (Pinelli and Buchthal, 1951). If the nerve supplying an affected muscle is stimulated electrically at tetanic frequency, there is a progressive decrease in amplitude of the evoked potentials (Hodes, 1948). The explanation of this abnormal fatiguability is unknown, but it must be due to some form of block developing at the neuromuscular junction, and it has been suggested that this occurs as a result of impairment of synthesis of acetyl choline in the damaged neurones (Simpson,

1966). It may be that the occurrence of peripheral sprouting, so that the neurone becomes responsible for an enlarged population of muscle fibres, is also a relevant factor.

Nerve conduction velocity is generally normal, or nearly normal, in patients with poliomyelitis. Early reports (Hodes, 1949) suggested that conduction velocity might be slower than normal, but it is now clear that this is not generally the case, provided that care is taken to correct for the low temperature which may exist in a severely paretic limb (Johnson et al., 1960).

MOTOR NEURONE DISEASE

Motor neurone disease is a condition in which there is progressive weakness and wasting of affected muscles, which is associated with degeneration of motor neurones in the brain and spinal cord. The two principal clinical varieties are referred to as amyotrophic lateral sclerosis and progressive muscular atrophy. In the latter variety, the process appears to be confined to the motor nerve cells, whereas in the former there is also degeneration of the corticospinal tracts giving rise to a combination of upper and lower motor neurone signs. The pathogenesis is at present unknown. Although normally only a small proportion of patients appear to have affected relatives, a variant of the disorder exists among the Chamorras in the Mariana Islands, which accounts for 10 per cent of the total mortality in the population. Clinically, the onset is frequently associated with the appearance of wasting of the small muscles of the hands, and widespread fasciculation may be an early feature. In some instances, weakness may start in the lower limb muscles or in the bulbar muscles, which are frequently affected in the later stages of the disease. Important conditions that give rise to diagnostic difficulty are cervical spondylosis, where secondary vascular changes may give rise to anterior horn cell damage in the cervical cord, peripheral neuropathy, particularly if sensory changes are not conspicuous, carcinomatous neuropathy, diabetic amyotrophy, and sometimes myasthenia gravis. Electromyography is frequently helpful in distinguishing motor neurone disease from these conditions. Particularly helpful may be the demonstration of widespread lower motor neurone involvement which is not consistent with a localised cervical lesion, or a disorder such as myasthenia gravis. The demonstration of a myelopathic motor neurone discharge pattern, in association with normal nerve conduction measurements, may distinguish motor neurone disease from a peripheral neuropathy. The electromyographic features of motor neurone disease are, in many respects, similar to those seen in poliomyelitis. Differences that occur are probably related to the steadily progressive character of motor neurone disease, in which anterior horn cell destruction continues throughout the course of the disease, in contrast to poliomyelitis where the nerve cell damage occurs during a short space of time in the acute stage. In both conditions there is diminished recruitment of motor unit potentials, which may be of increased amplitude and duration and may be recorded synchronously from different parts of affected muscle. Fasciculation is a more prominent feature of motor neurone disease than poliomyelitis. In poliomyelitis the integrated electromyogram may show very high mean voltages at low tensions, whereas in motor neurone disease the mean voltage at a given tension is similar to that recorded in healthy muscle (Lenman, 1959).

Spontaneous activity at rest, in the form of fibrillation and positive sharp waves together with an excess of insertion activity, is common in motor neurone disease, but fibrillation may be less conspicuous than might be anticipated from the degree of wasting. Fasciculation is frequently conspicuous and large. Sometimes polyphasic potentials occurring apparently spontaneously are recorded in relaxed muscle. Although in advanced motor neurone disease, where there is marked weakness and wasting, and electrical signs of partial denervation may be present, there may be little difficulty in assessing the significance of fasciculation. It is frequently a matter of difficulty to differentiate the fasciculations of possible motor neurone disease from those which are seen in patients with root or peripheral nerve lesions, or even in healthy individuals. The characteristics of individual fasciculation potentials are in no way specific, but Trojaborg and Buchthal (1965) have suggested that the frequency of firing may be of some value, the fasciculations of motor neurone disease appearing at a slower rate, about 3/10 seconds, compared with the fasciculations of other conditions which appear at a frequency often exceeding 1 a second.

The motor unit pattern seen on voluntary effort in motor neurone disease is the characteristic one of spinal muscular atrophy. There is a diminished or absent interference pattern, with motor unit action potentials of high amplitude and abnormally long duration appearing as discrete units even on maximal effort. In advanced cases, where only a few potentials can be recorded, the potentials may be seen to be occurring rapidly at about 50 a second, even during a comparatively weak contraction, indicating that this represents practically maximum effort (Willison, 1962). During voluntary contraction in severely affected muscles, individual motor units frequently show a rapid fall in amplitude and, if the motor nerve to a weak muscle is tetanised, there may be a rapid decrement in the evoked potential (Mulder et al., 1959; Simpson and Lenman, 1959; see also Chapter 11).

Motor and sensory nerve conduction velocity are usually only slightly impaired. In severely affected patients the evoked potentials, following motor nerve stimulation, may be greatly reduced in amplitude and sometimes, when only a few motor nerve fibres survive in the nerve trunks, it may be difficult or impossible to record any evoked potential. When the limbs are extremely weak they are frequently cold, and adequate temperature control is particularly important when carrying out conduction velocity studies on these patients. The continued persistence of a sensory nerve action potential in cases where the motor fibres of a nerve have all undergone degeneration is sometimes of value in distinguishing the condition from diabetic amyotrophy, where sensory nerve action potentials are frequently also lost (Willison, 1962).

CERVICAL SPONDYLOSIS

In cervical spondylosis, where the neurological deficit is associated with degenerative disease of the cervical spine, several mechanisms may give rise to muscular weakness and wasting. Compression of nerve roots by osteophytes may lead to weakness and wasting, which has a characteristically segmental distribution. Fasciculation is sometimes present, but less regularly than is the case in anterior horn cell disease. Exploration of an affected muscle with a concentric electrode may show evidence of partial denervation in the form of excessive insertion activity, fibrillation potentials, and positive sharp waves. On voluntary activity, there may be reduced motor unit activity with motor unit action potentials of normal or increased duration. Although there may be some excess of polyphasic units, the high amplitude units seen in motor neurone disease are not characteristic.

Motor nerve conduction velocity measurement usually shows no significant abnormality. This is because peripheral nerves, which are accessible to nerve conduction velocity measurement, generally receive motor fibres arising from several roots so that, even if a single root is wholly destroyed, fast conducting fibres from another root are available to transmit the nerve impulse with a normal latency. Conduction along sensory nerves is also generally unimpaired. Compression of a cervical root by a disc or by an osteophyte will affect it central to the posterior root ganglion and, hence, will not cause degeneration along the peripheral fibres of the sensory nerve. In a brachial plexus lesion, on the other hand, loss of sensory nerve potentials may be an early finding.

Myelopathy is a fairly frequent feature of cervical spondylosis, and may result from direct pressure on the cord by a displaced disc or by an osteophyte, or occur through interference with the blood supply to the cord. In the latter instance, there may be degeneration of the anterior horn cells and, here, the electromyographic changes in the affected segments may be indistinguishable from those of motor neurone disease. The distribution of the abnormality is of particular value because, in cervical spondylosis, the electromyographic evidence of a lower motor neurone lesion is generally confined to a few adjacent segments, whereas in motor neurone disease it may be widespread and involve both upper and lower extremities.

SYRINGOMYELIA

The electromyographic changes here are indistinguishable from those seen in any intramedullary tumour, and are principally due to pressure on anterior horn cells. As such, they are indistinguishable from those of motor neurone disease, although usually localised to relatively few spinal segments. Patients with syringomyelia frequently have severe spondylotic changes in the cervical spine at a relatively early age, and in this event may also show features of radiculopathy.

The Peripheral Neuropathies

In the investigation of patients with peripheral neuropathy, nerve conduction velocity measurement adds greatly to the clinical value of electromyography. In the clinical analysis of muscular weakness, the character of the motor unit action potentials will frequently make it possible to distinguish a myopathy from a neuropathy.

In some instances, the presence of electrical signs of denervation will show that weakness is due to a lower motor neurone lesion, rather than a disorder of the white matter in the brain or spinal cord. On the other hand, the polyphasic units seen in some cases of peripheral neuropathy may be difficult to differentiate from the units seen in muscular dystrophy, and the presence of fibrillation and positive sharp waves in polymyositis may be misinterpreted as providing evidence of a neuropathy. The finding of a substantial slowing of nerve conduction velocity is strong evidence of pathology affecting a peripheral nerve. On the other hand, not all cases of peripheral neuropathy show reduction in conduction velocity, so that whereas impairment of nerve conduction velocity is always a significant finding, the recording of normal values must be interpreted with caution and in the light of other methods of study.

ELECTROMYOGRAPHY IN PERIPHERAL NEUROPATHY

The most characteristic electromyographic finding in peripheral neuropathy is a reduction in motor unit activity, so that in severe weakness individual units can be clearly identified even during maximal effort, so that the interference pattern is lost or markedly reduced. The motor unit action potentials are frequently polyphasic, probably due to impairment of conduction velocity in the fine terminal branches of the nerves which innervate the fibres comprising the motor units. This excess of polyphasic units, which may be associated with a shift to the high frequency end of the spectrum if automatic frequency analysis is carried out may lead to confusion with myopathic weakness, although in myopathies there is generally a full, or nearly full, interference pattern on maximum effort, even in the presence of severe weakness. Measurement of the action potential dimensions in peripheral neuropathy has shown the amplitude of the potentials to be either normal or slightly diminished; the mean action potential duration is likewise normal, or may be slightly increased (Buchthal and Pinelli, 1953).

The presence of signs of denervation is variable. In an acute peripheral neuritis, fibrillation and positive sharp waves are not usually seen until several weeks after the onset. Eventually, they may occur profusely but in some cases may be difficult to find even when weakness is severe, possibly indicating that the pathological process has been one in which segmental demyelination has been the predominant feature with relatively minor changes in the axons. The presence of fibrillation is of assistance in assessing prognosis, because when it is present in profusion it indicates that Wallerian degeneration of the nerve supplying the muscle has taken place, so that recovery can come about only through the relatively lengthy process of regeneration.

NERVE CONDUCTION MEASUREMENT IN PERIPHERAL NEUROPATHY

Conduction velocity measurements in both motor and sensory nerves may be of considerable assistance in the study of peripheral neuropathies. In both motor and sensory nerve conduction studies, an absolute fall in conduction velocity compared with normal may be found. In motor nerve conduction studies, the evoked muscle action potential, even if it has a normal latency, may be of extended duration with an abnormal number of phases. In sensory nerve studies, the action potential may be of very much reduced amplitude or may be unobtainable.

The two most important factors which determine nerve conduction velocity are nerve fibre diameter, and whether or not the nerve fibre has an intact myelin sheath. Generally speaking, the conduction velocity of mammalian nerve fibres depends on fibre size, the fibres of largest diameter having the most rapid conduction velocity. In myelinated nerve fibres, conduction is saltatory, i.e. the nerve impulse is transmitted as a change in potential spreading from one node of Ranvier to the next, through the electrolyte medium surrounding the nerve fibres. Since passage of the impulse in this way is much more rapid than is the spread of depolarisation along the nerve fibre membrane, myelinated nerves conduct their impulses more rapidly than unmyelinated fibres. A third factor, which might be expected to affect nerve conduction velocity, is the distance apart of the nodes of Ranvier, but in practice this seems to have little effect. After nerve conduction velocity has become stabilised in early childhood, internodal distance continues to increase with growth of the limbs, without any corresponding increase in conduction velocity (Gilliatt, 1966). Degeneration of the axon itself has relatively little effect on nerve conduction velocity—apparently, provided an axon with intact myelin sheath is able to conduct an impulse at all, it does so at its maximum velocity.

Two mechanisms, therefore, might seem to be involved in impairment of nerve conduction velocity; one is the selective destruction of large nerve fibres, so that only the smaller, more slowly conducting fibres remain to conduct impulses; the second is demyelination of the nerves, so that saltatory conduction is affected. The second mechanism is the more important, but the first may account for some of the cases where anterior horn cell disease is associated with conduction velocities which, by a small margin, lie outside the normal range. Demyelination can occur, apparently as a primary change, with little corresponding involvement of the axon, and there is evidence that this may occur in those neuropathies where slowing of conduction velocity is a regular and conspicuous finding. When Wallerian degeneration occurs secondary to nerve trauma or degeneration of the nerve cell, demyelination also occurs but it is a less conspicuous feature until an advanced stage is reached, the damage mainly affecting the axon. In Wallerian degeneration conduction velocity is frequently affected, but it is seldom reduced by more than 30 per cent.

Examples of individual neuropathies will be considered below. The evidence at present available suggests that peripheral neuropathy can be divided into two large groups. In the first, the neurone appears to be primarily affected and the changes in the nerve fibres are those of secondary Wallerian degeneration. This group includes many of the nutritional and toxic neuropathies, and probably the neuropathy associated with porphyria. In the second group, there is segmental demyelination which, in some cases, may be related to changes occurring in the Schwann cells. In this group, conduction velocity may be slowed by more than 40 per cent, and important examples are the Guillain-Barré syndrome and the neuropathies associated with diphtheria, diabetes, and carcinoma (Gilliatt, 1966).

ACUTE 'INFECTIVE' POLYNEURITIS—
GUILLAIN-BARRÉ SYNDROME

The nature of this syndrome remains uncertain, but the failure to isolate any infective agent, the similarity of many of its features to experimental allergic neuropathy following injection of nerve tissue, along with an adjuvant, and the apparent clinical response of some cases to steroid therapy, suggests that it may represent an allergic reaction, possibly to a preceding infection. Pathologically, there is segmental demyelination which is frequently most pronounced proximally in the nerve roots.

The electromyographic changes follow the typical pattern of a peripheral neuropathy. In the acute stage the only abnormality may be reduction of motor unit activity or, in severely affected muscles, electrical silence. After three to four weeks, fibrillation may be seen but it is not infrequently scanty. In the later stages, and as recovery takes place, polyphasic units make their appearance.

Changes in nerve conduction velocity may occur both in acute and chronic forms of the illness, and when they occur they may be very marked, with velocities sometimes as low as 10 m/sec (Lambert, 1962). The reason why conduction velocity should be normal in some cases is not clear, but it may be related to the demyelination occurring proximally, so that conduction in the distal segments of the nerves is relatively unaffected. Conduction velocity measurement is particularly valuable in children with this disorder, the more so in cases where there is little or no sensory disturbance, and the condition clinically may resemble a myopathy. Nerve conduction measurement using surface electrodes causes little distress and, if marked slowing of nerve conduction is found, it is virtually diagnostic. When nerve conduction velocity is slowed, the slowing is generally present diffusely along the course of the nerves, but sometimes it is most prominent at common sites of nerve compression (Lambert and Mulder, 1963).

DIABETIC NEUROPATHY

While diabetic neuropathy is frequently asymmetrical in distribution, and may effect the nerve supply predominantly of a single limb, or even present as a mononeuritis, an acute polyneuritis may occur, which is mainly sensory in character, symmetrical in distribution, and frequently associated with severe autonomic disturbances. In the variety known as diabetic amyotrophy, the predominant feature is proximal muscular weakness, with little sensory involvement and often affecting particularly the quadriceps femoris. Many patients with diabetes show no symptoms of neuropathy, but on examination vibration sense is lost below the knees and the ankle jerks cannot be obtained.

The pathogenesis of diabetic neuropathy is unknown. It is not necessarily associated with poor control of diabetes and it is not uncommon for diabetic polyneuropathy to be the first clinical manifestation of the disease. On the other hand, both diabetic polyneuropathy and diabetic amyotrophy may improve considerably with strict control of the diabetes. It is also uncertain how far the neuropathy is related to ischaemic changes in the nerve fibres, or to a metabolic change in the peripheral nerve. Probably the latter is more important (Greenbaum et al., 1964), although the prevalence of neuropathy at common sites of nerve compression (see Fig. 7.2) suggests that the nerves in diabetes are particularly vulnerable to ischaemia (Simpson, 1962). Thomas and Lascelles (1965) have demonstrated segmental demyelination in teased-out single nerve fibres, and suggest that the primary metabolic change may lie in the Schwann cells.

The electromyographic changes in diabetic neuropathy are in no way specific, representing those seen commonly in peripheral neuropathy. Strength duration curves commonly show discontinuities (Greenbaum, 1964). A prominent feature may be a reduction in motor unit activity with some increase in polyphasic potentials, and in mean action potential duration. Fibrillation may be scanty and this may be because the peripheral ischaemia, which is associated with diabetes, may give rise to low intramuscular temperatures (Buchthal, 1966). Another factor may be that many of the axons remain intact in a process which predominantly may affect the myelin sheath.

Conduction velocity measurement is of particular interest in diabetes. It is clear that not only may all forms of diabetic neuropathy show slowing of nerve conduction velocity, but also that patients with diabetes, who have no clinical symptoms of neuropathy may show slowing of conduction (Mulder et al., 1961; Lawrence and Locke, 1961; Downie and Newell, 1961). Moreover, patients who have what is clinically a sensory neuropathy may have substantial slowing of conduction velocity in motor nerves. In these patients, a significant abnormality is reduction in size or even loss of evoked nerve action potentials in both lower and upper limbs (Gilliatt and Willison, 1962; Downie, 1964). While in many cases impairment of nerve conduction velocity is widespread, it is not uncommonly asymmetrical, and in some instances of isolated mononeuritis it can only be demonstrated in the clinically affected nerve. This would favour in these instances a local ischaemic effect on a nerve exposed to abnormal pressure. On the other hand, the observation that in cases of polyneuropathy where motor nerve conduction is affected the velocity may be slowed to as little as 10 m/sec, suggests that in these cases segmental demyelination following a metabolic change in the Schwann cells may be the operative mechanism.

In the syndrome of diabetic amyotrophy, the finding of impaired motor nerve conduction velocity is of particular value in differentiating the condition from myelopathy due to cord compression, or a spinal muscular atrophy such as motor neurone disease.

TOXIC, NUTRITIONAL, AND METABOLIC NEUROPATHY

This group includes neuropathies due to known chemical poisons such as lead, arsenic, and tri-ortho-cresyl phosphate, to drugs such as thalidomide, nitrofurantoin, and isonicotinic hydrazide, and to the exotoxin of C. diphtheriae. Nutritional disorders that may give rise to neuropathy are beri-beri, pellagra, and vitamin B12 neuropathy, and it is likely that alcoholic neuropathy is also a nutritional rather than a toxic disorder. Porphyria, particularly the acute intermittent form, is an example of a genetically determined metabolic disorder that may be associated with an acute polyneuropathy. The neuropathy associated with uraemia may be a toxic manifestation, although nothing is known about the toxic substances which may be involved. The neuropathy associated with carcinoma is probably a metabolic disorder, although nothing is at present known about the nature of the underlying disturbance.

In many of these neuropathies, the diagnosis of neuropathy can be determined quite readily on clinical grounds. Determination of the cause of the neuropathy may involve detailed clinical and biochemical study, and electromyography and nerve conduction study may have a limited value in distinguishing one variety from another. The majority of the toxic neuropathies are due to a primary change in the neurone, with secondary changes in the axon, and ultimate Wallerian degeneration. Exceptions are lead neuropathy and diphtheritic neuropathy, in which segmental demyelination seems to be the primary change. In all these types of neuropathy, electromyography may show evidence of lower motor neurone involvement in varying degree. In the predominantly motor neuropathy of tri-ortho-cresyl phosphate intoxication, and in the sensory-motor neuropathies due to thalidomide, nitrofurantoin and isoniazid motor nerve conduction velocity is frequently within, or close to, the normal range and this is also the case in porphyria (Simpson, 1962; Gilliatt, 1966).

In early cases of lead poisoning motor nerve conduction velocity may be normal but measurement and comparison of the amplitude of the evoked muscle potential following stimulation at different sites along the nerve may show abnormalities. If conduction is slowed in a few fibres of the nerve there may be sufficient temporal disperson following stimulation at a site distant from the muscle to lead to significant reduction in the size of the evoked potential. The ratio of amplitude between the potential evoked by proximal to that evoked by distal stimulation may therefore be a sensitive sign of a developing neuropathy (Fullerton, 1969).

In the neuropathy which is sometimes associated with carcinoma, conduction quite frequently shows fairly marked slowing. In alcoholic neuropathy there may be moderate slowing of conduction velocity, but this seldom exceeds 30 per cent (Mawdsley and Mayer, 1965). Slowing of conduction velocity is a frequent finding in uraemic neuropathy. In severe cases slowing may be very marked, and moderate degrees of slowing may occur in uraemic patients who do not show clinical evidence of neuropathy (Stewart *et al.*, 1968; Lenman, 1968).

INTERSTITIAL NEURITIS
In certain of the connective tissue disorders a neuropathy may occur which, in some cases, is due to involvement of the supporting tissues of the nerves or of the vasa vasorum. Conditions where such a mechanism may be a factor are polyarteritis nodosa, disseminated lupus erythematosis, and rheumatoid arthritis, and in all these conditions there may be slowing of nerve conduction velocity as well as abnormalities in the electromyogram. In leprosy, the infective granulamatous process may involve the peripheral nerves, and electromyography may show evidence of partial denervation in the distribution of the affected peripheral nerves (Baccaredda-Boy *et al.*, 1963). Impairment of conduction velocity has also been described in leprosy, showing progressive improvement during clinical remission (Granger, 1966).

HEREDITARY NEUROPATHY
The commonest condition within this group is peroneal muscular atrophy or Charcot-Marie-Tooth disease. This is inherited as an

autosomal dominant, and in affected subjects there is a slowly progressive weakness and wasting of the limbs starting distally and spreading proximally to a strictly limited extent. Pes cavus is generally present, and sometimes there is peripheral impairment of touch and pinprick sensation. It is generally considered to be a form of spinal muscular atrophy with loss of anterior horn cells in restricted regions of the cord. However, the marked slowing of conduction velocity that may occur indicates that the peripheral nerves are also involved in the process. Haase and Shy (1960) have described myopathic as well as neuropathic changes in the affected muscles.

Electromyography, however, has shown no evidence of a myopathic process (Amick and Lemmi, 1963; Buchthal, 1965). Fibrillations may be present at rest, and on voluntary contraction there may be reduced motor unit activity with high amplitude units suggestive of a myelopathic process. Motor nerve conduction velocity is slowed in many, but not in all, affected patients, and minimal slowing has been recorded in the nerves of clinically healthy members of affected families. Very marked slowing, with velocities of less than 10 m/sec has occasionally been recorded (Amick and Lemmi, 1963; Myrianthopoulos et al., 1964).

In the hypertrophic polyneuritis of Dejerine and Sottas the peripheral nerves can be palpated as thickened structures, which histologically is due to the nerve being surrounded by lamellae of tissue, and individual teased out fibres show segmental demyelination. Conduction velocities as low as 3 m/sec have been recorded. In Refsum's disease, which is also recessive, there is an inborn error of lipid metabolism with deposits of phytanic acid in the tissues. The peripheral nerves show a hypertrophic neuropathy similar to that in Dejerine-Sottas disease, but there is also ichthyosis, cerebellar ataxia and atypical retinitis pigmentosa (Dyck and Lambert, 1968). These forms of hypertrophic polyneuropathy share with Charcot-Marie-Tooth disease the characteristic that the peripheral nerves show not only marked slowing of conduction velocity but frequently have an abnormally high threshold to electrical stimulation (Simpson, 1969).

Metachromatic leucodystrophy is a rare lipoidosis, but is of interest because metachromatic granules can be demonstrated within the Schwann cells, and the nerves show the marked slowing of conduction velocity which may be associated with segmental demyelination (Fullerton, 1964).

9

9
The Facial Nerve

The facial nerve is most frequently injured in that segment which lies in the bony canal within the petrous temporal bone. Here, it may be damaged by fractures of the temporal bone or exposed to compression by pus or granulation tissue, as in suppurative otitis media. It is this portion of the nerve which is usually affected in Bell's palsy, the commonest affection of the facial nerve. This is generally an isolated neuropathy which develops apparently spontaneously in an otherwise healthy person, but sometimes facial palsy may be a feature of a generalised neuritis. Within the cranial cavity the facial nerve may be compressed by tumour, such as an acoustic neuroma, and after it has left the skull it may be exposed to trauma near the stylo-mastoid foramen.

A number of cases of facial palsy are associated with an eruption in the internal auditory meatus, and on the anterior pillar of the fauces, and are due to herpes zoster affecting the geniculate ganglion. Since the cells of the first sensory neurone for taste lie in the geniculate ganglion, geniculate herpes is generally associated with loss of taste sensation in the anterior two thirds of the tongue, but loss of taste may occur in any condition where the facial nerve is affected above the point where the chorda tympani leaves it. The significance of loss of taste sensation in relation to the severity of the lesion is uncertain, but it has been suggested that in Bell's palsy impairment of taste sensation may be evidence of partial denervation. On the basis of this, a technique has been developed to measure the threshold of the tongue to taste by applying a small current of known intensity (less than 100 μA) to the surface of the tongue through the anode of a battery generator (Peiris and Miles, 1965).

In facial palsy the principal value of electrodiagnostic techniques is in the assessment of prognosis. Where the lesion is one of neurapraxia or simple conduction block (*see* Chapter 7) recovery is generally rapid and uncomplicated. On the other hand, if the continuity of the axon is interrupted, recovery is likely to be slow and may be incomplete.

114

In Bell's palsy many cases recover completely within a few weeks, and in more than half recovery is complete. In about 40 per cent of cases there is some degree of denervation, but it is only in about 15 per cent of the whole that the patient is left with no significant recovery of function (Taverner, 1959). In Bell's palsy electrodiagnosis is of considerable value in assigning patients to the appropriate prognostic category. In traumatic and compressive lesions of the nerve, the question of surgical treatment may depend on how far the continuity of the nerve has been interrupted, and this may be assessed most reliably by electrophysiological study. In the electrical examination of the facial nerve, the techniques which at present are of established value and include electromyography, nerve conduction measurement, and the study of the strength-duration relationship and accommodation.

ELECTROMYOGRAPHY AND NERVE CONDUCTION MEASUREMENT

Electromyography of the facial muscles may be carried out, using a fine concentric electrode to explore either the frontalis or the orbicularis oris muscles. Since the motor unit action potentials in the facial muscles are of relatively short duration compared with motor unit potentials recorded from the limb muscles (*see* Chapter 2), care must be taken to distinguish fibrillation from scanty voluntary motor unit activity.

If fibrillation is recorded, this indicates that a proportion of the muscle fibres have undergone denervation, so that electromyography may provide evidence of partial denervation. Fibrillation, however, may not appear until as much as three weeks have elapsed from the time of development of the nerve lesion, and it thus provides later information regarding the state of the nerve than either nerve-conduction measurement or the intensity-duration relationship. Electromyography is particularly useful when evidence of re-innervation is sought. Thus, if the face has been totally paralysed and no voluntary movement can be seen, the appearance of motor unit action potentials on electromyography may be the earliest sign that recovery is likely to take place.

Conduction in the facial nerve may be studied by measuring the terminal latency in the nerve after stimulation at the angle of the jaw. Stimulation may be carried out through surface electrodes, and evoked potentials can be recorded either from orbicularis oris or the frontalis muscle. In either situation recording may be carried out with a fine concentric needle electrode, but satisfactory evoked potentials can also be obtained if surface electrodes are used (Fig. 9.1). At the orbicularis oris it is less easy to obtain satisfactory contact between the electrodes and the skin. One arrangement which has been found suitable is to employ silver disc electrodes of the 'stick-on' variety used for electroencephalography. Another is to use

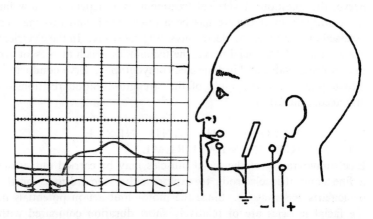

FIGURE 9.1 Action potential recorded with surface electrodes over orbicularis oris following stimulation of the facial nerve at the angle of the jaw. Oscilloscope sweep speed is 1 cm/s, so that the latency is less than 3 msec, which is normal. Silver discs, such as EEG stick-on electrodes, are suitable recording electrodes.

'clip-on' electrodes of the type described by Copland and Davies (1964).

Conduction measurement provides relatively early evidence of denervation since it has been shown that all conduction ceases in the distal segment of the nerve by the seventh day following nerve section (Gilliatt and Taylor, 1959). Failure to obtain an evoked potential during the second week after the development of a facial palsy is therefore strong evidence that denervation is complete. This conclusion, however, can only be reached if the technical arrangements are such that it is certain that failure to obtain an evoked potential is not due to technical factors. On the other hand, the presence of an evoked potential occurring after a normal latency is evidence that the nerve lesion may be no more than a neurapraxia. Where the conduction latency is prolonged, careful study during the succeeding weeks nearly always discloses fibrillation potentials, so that in practice a lengthened conduction latency is generally an indication of partial denervation; partial denervation of this order, however, is frequently associated with good functional recovery (Langworth and Tavener, 1963; Taverner, 1965).

In the early assessment of Bell's palsy, therefore, the presence of an evoked potential, with either a normal or prolonged latency during the second week, indicates a favourable prognosis in that there will certainly be partial recovery and probably complete recovery. If no evoked potential can be recorded, complete denervation is likely and the outlook is extremely doubtful. With trauma to the facial nerve the situation is less satisfactory, because it is important to know the state of the nerve as early as possible, but no test at present available will distinguish between neurapraxia and axonotmesis in less than seven days.

ELECTRICAL STIMULATION

The superficial position of the facial muscles renders them accessible to stimulation, and intensity-duration curves are of considerable value.

The sensitivity of the face, especially in apprehensive or young subjects, makes it essential to use a low-impedance stimulator, and the minor advantages of deep denervation detection by the high-impedance type are not significant. Evidence of partial denervation is often found within a few days of the onset of Bell's Palsy, even in cases where recovery takes place within a few weeks; but I-D curves typical of massive denervation imply that regeneration, if it occurs, will take several months and that recovery is unlikely to be complete. It is noteworthy that, in the facial muscles, denervation does not proceed to atrophy as rapidly as in muscles elsewhere, and contractile but totally denervated muscle has been detected by the I-D curve many years after the original lesion.

Accommodation measurement is of great value in assessing facial muscle denervation. The relative specificity of triangular pulses for denervated muscle as compared to normal allows identification with ease, and the procedure is well tolerated by the patient.

Changes in electrical excitability appear several weeks before clinical signs of re-innervation, the interval being as a rule more constant (6 to 9 weeks) than elsewhere, no doubt due to the relatively small bulk of the facial muscles and the greater likelihood of detection of minor amounts of denervation.

10
Diseases of Muscle

Diseases of muscle include a genetically determined group of disorders known as the muscular dystrophies, acquired myopathies which include the polymyositis syndrome and various endocrine myopathies and a miscellaneous group of congenital disorders. An important group of diseases are those in which myotonia is a predominant symptom.

In all these conditions there is no demonstrable pathology in the central or peripheral nervous system. The electromyographic abnormalities depend on the fact that, while, in general, the number of motor units activated is normal, the motor units themselves show abnormalities which give rise to abnormal electrical appearances. This may arise because the structure of the motor units is modified through loss of some of the constituent fibres, so that the motor unit potentials have abnormal characteristics. In addition, in many myopathic conditions the membrane properties of the individual fibres are altered, and this gives rise to changes in excitability which can be recognised electromyographically.

While these changes are of considerable value in assisting diagnosis, they require careful interpretation. The motor unit characteristics seen in disordered muscle must be distinguished from those which indicate abnormal innervation. The characteristic electromyographic feature of myopathy is the polyphasic motor unit action potential, which is seen when some of the fibres comprising the motor unit have been lost, and the remaining fibres give rise to separate recognisable spikes because they are not contracting synchronously. However, in peripheral neuropathy there may be impairment of conduction velocity in the distal nerve terminals, so that some of the fibres are activated after a delay which leads to dispersal of the potentials of the individual fibres, and the whole unit potential becomes polyphasic. On the other hand, in neuropathy there is usually a reduction in the number of motor units activated during a strong contraction, so that the interference pattern is reduced or even lost altogether. In the myopathies, the interference pattern is generally well maintained up to a late stage in the disease. The excitability changes in the muscle fibres in certain varieties of myopathy may also give rise to difficulty, since fibrillation potentials and abnormal insertion activity, when they occur in myopathy, may be confused with the appearance seen in partial denervation. Here again, the presence of a full, or nearly full, interference pattern in myopathy, together with the absence of any alteration in nerve conduction velocity are useful distinguishing features.

In order to try to establish specific diagnostic criteria, and also to detect the minor abnormalities seen in mildly affected patients, a number of methods for analysing the electromyogram quantitatively have been developed (*see* Chapter 3). The observation that clinically unaffected carriers of muscular dystrophy may have minor abnormalities in the electromyogram has added interest to these techniques. Important methods which have been developed include the measurement of mean action potential duration, automatic frequency analysis, the study of integrated electrical activity and its relationship to tension, spike counting techniques, and refractory period measurement. In this chapter, the electromyographic changes which occur in muscular dystrophy will first be discussed in some detail. In later sections the findings in other disorders of muscle will be considered.

MUSCULAR DYSTROPHY

CLASSIFICATION OF MUSCULAR DYSTROPHY

Although early attempts at classification of muscular dystrophy relied mainly on clinical description, it has gradually become possible to develop a classification based on genetic criteria, which is of value in giving prognostic guidance in individual cases. The current accepted classification is derived from that put forward by Walton and Natrass in 1954 and subsequently modified (Walton, 1964; Walton and Gardner-Medwin, 1968). In this classification muscular dystrophy is divided into three categories according to mode of inheritance. The first is the X-linked variety, in which the gene is carried on the X chromosome and the disease is transmitted by females and occurs in males. This category includes the common severe (Duchenne) form and the less common mild (Becker) variety. The second category is transmitted as an autosomal recessive, and includes a large heterogeneous group known as the limb-girdle variety and an uncommon group which resembles the Duchenne variety. The third category is transmitted as an autosomal dominant and includes the common facio-scapulo-humeral (Landouzy-Dejerine) variety, the rare distal variety, and the ocular myopathies.

While the majority of cases fall into this classification, sporadic cases without family history are not uncommon, and exceptional cases occur in which the mode of inheritance does not fall into the usual pattern. Thus, cases of limb-girdle dystrophy are sometimes seen in which the mode of inheritance is dominant.

SPONTANEOUS ELECTRICAL ACTIVITY

Although spontaneous activity has been described as occurring in hereditary forms of muscular dystrophy (Buchthal and Rosenfalck, 1963), it is comparatively uncommon in this form of muscle disease, in contrast to polymyositis where it occurs relatively frequently. Spontaneous activity, when it occurs, may take the form of brief discharges of repetitive activity following insertion or movement of the electrode and of fibrillation potentials. Norris and Chatfield (1955) have described this form of activity as particularly liable to occur after a powerful voluntary contraction.

THE MOTOR UNIT ACTION POTENTIAL

While a muscle in a patient with muscular dystrophy may give rise to large numbers of motor unit action potentials which are of normal shape, amplitude, and duration, careful exploration of affected muscles will generally reveal an excess of polyphasic units containing five or more phases (Kugelberg, 1949). These potentials arise because the electrode is recording near a unit or a subunit which has lost a proportion of its fibres, and the remaining fibres give rise to potentials which do not occur synchronously and therefore appear as separate spikes. Polyphasic units are most easily recognised by visual inspection of the oscilloscope screen (see Plate 7B) and when fed into a loudspeaker they give rise to a characteristic noise which assists in identifying them. Frequently, a muscle needs to be explored through a considerable proportion of its volume to find abnormal potentials. On account of this, and because polyphasic potentials also occur with varying frequency in healthy muscle, considerable experience may be necessary to decide whether these potentials, if they occur relatively sparsely, constitute a significant abnormality. It is for this reason that quantitative methods of analysis may be of value in the study of borderline cases. Another feature of myopathic muscle is that it is frequently infiltrated with fatty tissue, and this may give rise to areas of relative electrical silence which are sometimes encountered as the muscle is explored. Measurement of the duration of the action potentials (*see* Chapter 3) shows that on the average they are of shorter duration than is the case in healthy muscle (Kugelberg, 1947, 1949). This reduction in action potential duration is probably related to the reduced number of fibres that the units contain (Buchthal *et al.*, 1960). Whether the action potentials of single fibres in human muscular dystrophy are of shorter duration than those of healthy muscle is not known. Although a large number of patients with muscular dystrophy show a decrease in the mean duration of the action potentials, in a substantial number of cases the mean duration may come within normal limits (Pinelli and Buchthal, 1953). Measurement of action potential duration is therefore of value if the distribution of potentials is abnormal. A normal histogram, however, does not exclude muscular dystrophy.

The voltage of individual motor units in muscular dystrophy is usually normal or slightly diminished. Voltage measurements in electromyography, however, are particularly variable and liable to be modified by recording technique, and this measurement is therefore of relatively little diagnostic value in muscular dystrophy.

THE INTERFERENCE PATTERN

Since there is no significant reduction in the number of motor units activated during voluntary contraction in muscular dystrophy, a full interference pattern is generally obtained on maximal effort. The characteristics of the interference pattern, however, may be abnormal in certain respects. First, there may be a slight but significant reduction in amplitude (Kugelberg, 1947, 1949). Second, the broken up character of the units giving rise to the interference pattern may present an abnormally spiky appearance on the cathode-ray tube, and a crackling sound on the loudspeaker. In muscles which are severely affected, the disproportion between the degree of weakness and the comparative reduction in the interference pattern may provide strong evidence of a myopathic process.

The interference pattern in muscular dystrophy may be studied quantitatively in various ways (*see* Chapter 3). The simplest is the method of automatic frequency analysis, which enables the frequency distribution of the electromyogram to be displayed in the form of a histogram on the oscilloscope screen (see Plates 9, 10 and 11). In patients with myopathy there may be a shift toward the higher frequencies, with the dominant frequency at the upper end of the spectrum (Richardson, 1951; Walton, 1952). Although this is a useful adjunct to the visual interpretation of the electromyogram, a sustained shift in the frequency analysis is seldom present in the absence of a recognisable excess of polyphasic units.

Other methods of analysis depend on recording the isometric tension of a muscle simultaneously with the electromyogram. Thus, if the integrated mean voltage of the electromyogram is plotted graphically against the tension, a linear relationship is obtained (Lippold, 1952). In muscular dystrophy the slope of the curve may be altered, so that the mean voltage at a given tension is higher than in healthy muscle (Lenman, 1959). Another approach is to count the total number of spikes in a segment of the interference pattern recorded at a constant tension. When this is done, it is found that higher spike counts are recorded in myopathic than in healthy muscle (Willison, 1964). The counting may be done electronically, and a further refinement is to analyse the results by computer so that the intervals between the spikes can also be measured and the distribution plotted. The interval between spikes tends to be shorter in muscular dystrophy, and determining the distribution of spike intervals in this way renders the analysis more specific (Willison, 1968).

EXCITABILITY CHANGES

While abnormal sensitivity to mechanical stimulation in the form of abnormal insertion activity is occasionally seen in muscular dystrophy, changes in excitability are not as a rule demonstrated by standard techniques. Measurement of refractory period, however, can be carried out by stimulating small groups of muscle fibres with paired pulses (see Chapter 3). In muscular dystrophy, the absolute refractory period has been found to be about 30 per cent shorter than in healthy muscle (Farmer et al., 1959). The refractory period is also shortened in some healthy carriers of Duchenne muscular dystrophy (Caruso and Buchthal, 1965). Although the study of refractory period is technically troublesome, it is of interest because it depends on the recovery time of the muscle fibre after it has been depolarised (Buchthal and Engbaek, 1963), and is, therefore, one method of studying the membrane properties of muscle fibres.

CLINICAL VARIETIES OF DYSTROPHY

It is not at present possible to differentiate the clinical varieties of muscular dystrophy from each other by electrodiagnostic methods. The principal value of electromyography is to differentiate muscular dystrophy from neuropathic disorders with which it may be confused. Recently, this has assumed particular importance in connection with the X-linked varieties, since genetic counselling is vitiated if the diagnosis of dystrophy is incorrectly made. It has become evident that a significant number of cases previously considered to have X-linked dystrophy, suffer from spinal muscular atrophy of the variety described by Kugelberg and Welander (1956).

In the majority of instances of muscular dystrophy studied, the technique of visual and auditory analysis of motor unit potentials, perhaps supplemented by automatic frequency analysis, is adequate to establish or confirm the diagnosis. The more specialised techniques of quantitative analysis are of considerable interest in connection with research, and their clinical place at present lies in the study of difficult and atypical cases, and in connection with carrier detection.

CARRIER DETECTION

In the X-linked varieties of muscular dystrophy, abnormalities have been recorded in the electromyogram in the muscles of clinically unaffected carriers of the disease. This finding is of particular interest since it has been found that some, but not all, carriers can be identified by alterations in the serum enzymes and in muscle histology. It seems possible that electromyography may increase the proportion of carriers that may be identified by laboratory methods.

It was originally noted that, if electromyography was carried out using visual analysis of the interference pattern and automatic frequency analysis to study the electromyogram, a certain proportion of carriers showed abnormalities (Barwick, 1963). This method, however, is relatively insensitive when it is necessary to decide whether minor changes represent a significant deviation from the normal, and possible quantitative methods have been intensively studied (Van den Bosch, 1963; Caruso and Buchthal, 1965; Willison, 1968; Gardner-Medwin, 1968). At present, no method has been shown to be of more than limited value, but it is of interest that clinically healthy carriers may differ from normal subjects in that the refractory period of the muscle fibres is, on average, shorter (Caruso and Buchthal, 1965). In addition, both the mean action potential duration (Gardner-Medwin, 1968) and the mean interval between the spikes of the interference pattern (Willison, 1968) may be reduced. The practical application of these observations presents considerable problems, but they suggest that electromyography may contribute to the problem of carrier detection along with biochemical and other methods.

POLYMYOSITIS

The polymyositis syndrome includes a group of disorders in which there is muscular weakness, which is frequently associated with signs of a more widespread connective tissue disorder. The suggestion has been put forward that the muscular weakness may be associated with involvement of the fine nerve terminals—'a neuromyositis'—(Bauwens, 1956), but this has not been definitely established. Walton and Adams (1958) have classified the clinical varieties into four main groups. In the first, there are muscular changes without involvement of the skin. In the second group, skin changes are a feature, although the muscular weakness is again the dominant characteristic and, here, the term dermatomyositis may be appropriate. In the third group, muscle changes occur as a feature of a predominantly connective tissue disorder, such as disseminated lupus or scleroderma. In the fourth group, polymyositis occurs in association with malignant disease.

The electromyographic changes are similar in the different varieties. During voluntary contraction the changes may be indistinguishable from those in muscular dystrophy. There is an interference pattern on maximal effort, an excess of polyphasic units, and the mean potential duration is significantly reduced (Buchthal and Pinelli, 1953). A frequent finding is that the changes are patchy in distribution, so that exploration of a muscle may reveal foci of abnormality surrounded by regions where the motor unit pattern is comparatively normal. One value of electromyography is that it provides a means to search muscles for areas of abnormality, and in this way define suitable sites for muscle biopsy.

An important distinguishing feature of polymyositis in comparison with muscular dystrophy, is that spontaneous electrical activity is a frequent feature in polymyositis. This takes the form of fibrillation potentials and positive saw-tooth potentials which occur in resting muscle, and a marked excess of insertion activity in response to electrode movement. This consists of bursts of short duration potentials, which resemble discharges seen in myotonia, but are of shorter duration and lesser intensity. Sometimes high frequency potentials occur, which are polyphasic and repeat at 10–150 a second, starting and stopping abruptly. It is not known whether this spontaneous activity is the result of partial denervation resulting from involvement of the fine nerve terminals (Bauwens, 1956; Richardson, 1956), or of altered excitability of the cell membrane (Buchthal and Rosenfalck, 1963). Denny-Brown (1960) has suggested that muscle necrosis may isolate part of the fibre from the end-plate zone, so that fibrillation potentials occur in the isolated segment of the fibre.

In a number of cases of polymyositis abnormalities of neuromuscular conduction are seen, which can be demonstrated by repetitive stimulation of a muscle through its motor nerve. Sometimes the evoked potentials show a typical decremental response, resembling that seen in myasthenia gravis, and sometimes there is an incremental response resembling that which may occur in the carcinomatous myasthenia syndrome (Simpson and Lenman, 1959).

ENDOCRINE MYOPATHIES

Muscular weakness may occur in thyrotoxicosis, myxoedema, Cushing's syndrome, hypopituitarism, Addison's disease, and following the use of steroid hormones, particularly those containing fluoride in the 9-alpha position. In metabolic bone disease a proximal myopathy may occur, which is seen occasionally in hyperparathyroidism (Bischoff and Esslen, 1965), and more commonly in association with osteomalacia (Smith and Stern, 1967).

In thyrotoxicosis a chronic myopathy with muscle wasting and proximal weakness may develop, particularly in older patients. In these cases, electromyography shows the characteristic features of a myopathy, viz. an interference pattern on maximal effort, a reduction in mean action potential duration, and an excess of polyphasic units. Spontaneous electrical activity does not usually occur. Although severe myopathy, sufficient to give rise to disability, is uncommon, examination of patients with thyrotoxicosis, even in the absence of obvious muscular symptoms, will frequently reveal some loss of muscle power and significant abnormalities in the electromyogram. Generally, the electromyographic abnormalities show little relationship to the severity of the thyrotoxicosis. As a rule, the myopathy gradually recovers in the course of a few months, when the thyrotoxicosis is given treatment (Sanderson and Adey, 1952; Hed *et al.*, 1958; Havard *et al.*, 1963). Thyrotoxicosis is occasionally associated with myasthenia gravis and with periodic paralysis, and coexistence of one of these disorders may give rise to anomalous electromyographic findings. In the myopathy of Cushing's syndrome and in steroid myopathy, the electromyographic abnormalities closely resemble those seen in thyrotoxic myopathy.

In hypothyroidism a variety of muscular abnormalities occur. The contraction of a muscle in myxoedema is slow, and this gives rise to the useful clinical sign that the ankle jerk when recorded graphically shows a prolonged relaxation time, which is not associated with any abnormality of the electrical response (Lambert *et al.*, 1951). Occasionally, patients with myxoedema show the features of Hoffman's syndrome in which the muscles show hypertrophy, weakness, and an increased consistency on palpation, and show a slowness of movement which is sometimes associated with a local contraction following percussion, which may resemble myotonia. However, electromyography shows no abnormality and, in particular, there are not myotonic discharges (Wilson and Walton, 1959). A number of cases of hypothyroidism, however, show a proximal muscle weakness, clinically resembling that seen in thyrotoxic myopathy and in which the electromyogram shows an interference pattern on maximal effort, polyphasic units, reduced action potential duration, and no abnormal spontaneous activity at rest. Some of these patients show improvement in the muscles on treatment with thyroxine (Åström *et al.*, 1961).

METABOLIC MYOPATHIES

The expression metabolic myopathies refers to a rare group of muscular disorders which have been shown to have a specific underlying biochemical basis. In general, diagnosis depends on the clinical and biochemical findings, and electromyography plays a relatively small part in their recognition.

PERIODIC PARALYSIS

This includes a group of disorders in which transient paralysis is the principal clinical feature, and there is usually a profound electrolyte disturbance particularly affecting potassium. Three important varieties exist which may be distinguished according to whether the blood potassium is lowered, raised, or normal.

The hypokalaemic variety includes a familial form which is inherited as an autosomal dominant. Sporadic cases also occur and some of these may include cases of potassium depletion secondary to renal disease, and similar attacks may occur in cases of aldosteronism. There is an occasional association of periodic paralysis with

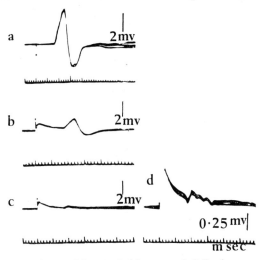

FIGURE 10.1 Evoked potentials recorded from muscle following nerve stimulation in a case of Periodic Paralysis. In (a) with a blood potassium level of 4·4 mEq/L the amplitude of the potential is 6·0 mV. There is a progressive reduction in amplitude with falls in blood potassium until at a potassium level of 1·8 mEq/L (c and d) the amplitude is 0·16 mV (*Courtesy of* J. A. Simpson).

thyrotoxicosis (Engel, 1961). The attacks of paralysis characteristically occur in the early morning, and consist of paralysis affecting the trunk and all four limbs, which may last for some hours. Electromyography during an attack shows the affected muscles to be electrically silent and unresponsive either to percussion or electrical stimulation (Fig. 10.1). In a mild attack there is a marked reduction of motor unit activity. It has been suggested that the paralysis may be due to hyperpolarisation of the muscle cells by migration of potassium into the muscle fibres during an attack, but the resting membrane potential has been measured during an attack and was not found to be raised (Shy *et al.*, 1961, *see also* Chapter 3).

A hyperkalaemic form of periodic paralysis has been termed adynamia episodica hereditaria by Gamstorp (1956). This condition is also transmitted as an autosomal dominant. The attacks which are associated with a high blood potassium, and are aggravated by potassium salts, generally occur during the day and are of relatively short duration. The condition may be associated with myotonia brought on particularly by cold, and a relationship with paramyotonia congenita has been postulated (Drager *et al.*, 1958). On electromyography there may be spontaneous potentials occurring at rest and these become more prominent during an attack, when there is reduced motor unit activity on voluntary contraction and many of the action potentials are of relatively short duration. Mechanical stimulation by electrode movement may be followed by excessive insertion activity and myotonic discharge (Buchthal *et al.*, 1958; Gamstorp, 1962). It has been suggested that during an attack there is a leakage of potassium from muscle cells, and this has received some support from the observation that the resting potential may be lowered (*see* Chapter 3) (Creutzfeldt *et al.*, 1963; McComas *et al.*, 1968).

A third type of periodic paralysis which resembles the hyperkalaemic form and is aggravated by potassium salts, but in which the blood potassium is normal has been described by Poskanzer and Kerr (1961).

MCARDLE'S SYNDROME

In this rare condition described by McArdle in 1951, pain and weakness occurs following muscular exercise. After exercise there is no rise in blood lactate or pyruvate, and the underlying biochemical abnormality has been shown to be a deficiency of muscle phosphorylase. Except in the presence of an attack, electromyography is usually normal. If, however, electromyography is carried out during ischaemic exercise of the forearm muscles, the muscles may be seen to go into contracture and in this state they are electrically silent.

MYOTONIA

Myotonia may occur in a number of syndromes, the most important of which are myotonia congenita (Thomsen's disease), dystrophia myotonica, paramyotonia congenita, myotonia paradoxa, and myotonia acquisita. Myotonia congenita is generally transmitted as an autosomal dominant and, as a rule, apart from some generalised hypertrophy of the muscles, myotonia constitutes the sole abnormality and the condition is compatible with a normal life span. In dystrophia myotonica the main disorder is a myopathy, and myotonia constitutes an additional feature. The myopathy affects the face, sternomastoids, and the muscles of the limbs with a characteristically distal distribution, and associated abnormalities include frontal baldness, cataract, and gonadal atrophy. The disease is transmitted as an autosomal dominant. In paramyotonia congenita, attacks are brought on by cold and may be followed by muscular weakness, and the condition is closely related to hyperkalaemic periodic paralysis (*vide supra*). Myotonia paradoxa is a variant of myotonia, in which the myotonia follows exercise in contrast to the commoner forms of myotonia which are relieved by exertion. Some cases of myotonia acquisita are probably atypical cases of dystrophia myotonica; others may be cases of hypothyroidism (Hoffmann's syndrome); and yet others are probably cases of neurogenic atrophy or polymyositis, in which electrical discharges resembling those of myotonia sometimes occur.

The two commonest varieties of myotonia are myotonia congenita and dystrophia myotonica. In both conditions the myotonic phenomenon is the same, although it is generally more severe in myotonia congenita. In dystrophia myotonica the typical electromyographic changes of a myopathy are present in the affected muscles, and are only distinguishable from those seen in muscular dystrophy by the additional presence of myotonia. In myotonia congenita the myotonic phenomena are the sole electromyographic abnormality.

Clinically, myotonia manifests itself by a delay in relaxation following a voluntary contraction, and by the appearance of muscular contraction after percussion. This contraction is seen as a slight depression under the skin and lasts for a few seconds. It should be distinguished from myoedema, which is a transient swelling of the muscle following percussion, which occurs occasionally in healthy people, frequently in cachectic states, and in hypothyroidism. In contrast to percussion myotonia, myoedema is electrically silent.

The electromyographic features of the myotonic reaction may be studied after a voluntary contraction, or following mechanical stimulation of the muscle, either by percussion or by movement of the exploring electrode. This gives rise to a high frequency discharge of potentials, in which the frequency gradually increases to reach a maximum of about 150 a second (*see* Chapter 2). This may be followed by a decrease both in amplitude and in frequency, which gives rise to the characteristic 'dive-bomber' sound on the loudspeaker. The potentials may be short duration, low amplitude potentials resembling those derived from single fibres; others are larger and have the character of motor unit potentials. Myotonic discharges likewise occur following a voluntary contraction, and when myotonic muscle is apparently relaxed short duration action potentials may occur, which have the appearance of being spontaneous. Whether these are wholly spontaneous or are evoked by minor degrees of movement is uncertain. They differ from fibrillation in that they are enhanced by a fall in temperature, which will usually bring fibrillation to an end (Buchthal and Rosenfalck, 1963).

The site of the abnormality in myotonia has been clearly shown to be peripheral, and probably lies in the muscle fibre membrane. Thus, the myotonic reaction is not abolished by curare either in man (Landau, 1952) or in the myotonic goat, where it persists after nerve section and end-plate degeneration (Brown and Harvey, 1939). It is abolished by substances which stabilise the muscle fibre membrane, such as quinine and procaine amide (Geschwind and Simpson, 1955). The resting membrane potential is probably normal in myotonia congenita, but it is reduced in dystrophia myotonica (*see* Chapter 3).

Discharges very similar to those which occur in myotonia, are occasionally seen in neurogenic muscular atophy and in polymyositis. These range from what is merely a moderate increase in insertion activity to discharges which are difficult to distinguish from those seen in myotonia, although they are generally less intense and less prolonged. High-frequency discharges of polyphasic units of abrupt onset and termination are sometimes evoked by electrode movement in polymyositis.

CONGENITAL MYOPATHIES
These include a group of rare conditions in which the diagnosis can be established precisely only by histological examination (Pearson *et al.*, 1967).

Arthrogryphosis multiplex congenita is a syndrome in which severe contractures and deformities of the limbs are present from birth. It does not represent a single disease entity, and many cases represent contractures associated with neurogenic atrophy. Some are instances of a congenital myopathy, and in these cases the electromyogram may show myopathic features.

Congenital myopathies which are clearly defined entities include central core disease, nemaline myopathy, the mitochondrial myopathies, and myotubular myopathy. Central core disease (Shy and Magee, 1956) is a rare congenital myopathy which is non-progressive, and in which histologically there is abnormality in the central region of the muscle fibres. Nemaline myopathy (Shy *et al.*, 1963) is likewise a non-progressive myopathy, which is inherited as an autosomal dominant. Histologically, the muscle fibres contain rod-shaped bodies lying under the sarcolemma, which appear to be composed of material identical with that of the Z-bands of the muscle fibres. In both central core disease and nemaline myopathy, the electromyogram may show a characteristic myopathic motor unit pattern.

Myotubular myopathy (Spiro *et al.*, 1966) is a rare disorder in which the affected muscles consist of persistent foetal myotubes, in which the central part of the fibre is devoid of myofibrils. In this condition the voluntary electromyogram may show a myopathic pattern, whereas the resting muscle may give rise to fibrillation potentials and myotonic discharges.

11
Myasthenia Gravis and Other Disorders of Neuromuscular Transmission

Although myasthenia gravis is the most important disease entity where the clinical defect is one of neuromuscular transmission, impairment of neuromuscular conduction may occur in a variety of circumstances. Thus, in polymyositis there may be abnormalities in neuromuscular transmission, and in the myasthenic syndrome, which is associated with carcinoma, neuromuscular conduction is impaired, but in a manner that differs in certain respects from what occurs in classical myasthenia. In patients with a severe neuropathy it is sometimes possible to demonstrate the presence of neuromuscular block, and many drugs and toxic agents are capable of modifying neuromuscular transmission. Electromyography has been of value in studying the physiology of neuromuscular transmission, and in clarifying the nature of the disturbance in disorders of neuromuscular transmission.

Under normal circumstances, conduction of the impulse from nerve to muscle is brought about by the liberation of acetyl choline from the nerve endings, which diffuses across the gap between nerve and muscle to bring about depolarisation of that part of the muscle fibre known as the end-plate zone. There is evidence that acetyl choline may be stored in submicroscopic bodies in the nerve fibre terminals known as 'synaptic vesicles'. Small quantities of acetyl choline are liberated continuously from the vesicles and give rise to small potentials at the end plate, which can be recorded with intra-cellular electrodes and which are known as miniature end-plate potentials. When a nerve impulse arrives at the nerve ending a substantial quantity of acetyl choline is released, possibly through disruption of a synaptic vesicle. How this comes about is not known, but one factor may be the entry of calcium ions into the presynaptic axoplasm during the action potential. Whereas calcium is necessary for the release of acetyl choline, magnesium ions and also procaine

132

and other local anaesthetics will reduce the amount of transmitter released.

When acetyl choline reaches the end-plate membrane of the muscle fibre, it reacts with end-plate receptors, and the effect of this is to short-circuit the polarised membrane at the end-plate by increasing the permeability to ions. An intracellular electrode will record the resulting end-plate potential, which in its turn activates the adjacent muscle membrane, giving rise to a propagated action potential which spreads along the muscle fibre. This action of acetyl choline is short-lived because it is inactivated by acetyl cholinesterase, which is present in the subneural apparatus underlying the end-plate membrane. Depolarisation is rapidly followed by the process of recovery or repolarisation, after which the muscle fibre is again ready to respond to a nerve impulse (Castillo and Katz, 1956).

The mechanism which couples the action potential with the chemical events of contraction is not understood, but there is evidence that calcium in some way activates the myosin in the A band of the muscle fibre (see Chapter 1) where the thick and thin filaments overlap, and initiates the tension generating reaction. Calcium may be sequestered within vesicles situated close to the myofibrils, and the release of calcium from these vesicles could be the critical event which sets off the contraction. The vesicles appear to communicate with the surface by transverse sarcoplasmic tubules, and it is possible that the action potential initiates an electrical change which passes along the tubules, and this has the effect of bringing about the release of calcium from the vesicles (Huxley, 1964).

Neuromuscular transmission may fail on account of disturbance, either within the nerve endings or at the motor end-plate, and the more important defects of transmission are as follows:

1. *Failure of transmitter synthesis.* This can be brought about by a group of substances known as hemicholiniums which inhibit the synthesis of acetyl choline. Neuromuscular block due to hemicholinium is characteristically slow in onset, since it is dependent on exhausting existing stores of acetyl choline. Because of this, block is accelerated by nerve stimulation and is related to its frequency.

2. *Failure of transmitter release.* Calcium ions are necessary for the release of ACh, and Mg ions reduce the amount of transmitter released. Botulinum toxin also blocks the release of ACh.

3. *Competitive block* may occur through the action of substances

which combine with the receptor for acetyl choline on the post-synaptic membrane to form an inactive complex. Tubocurarine and gallamine are important examples. The effect of tubocurarine is to cause a progressive reduction in amplitude of the end-plate potential, which eventually disappears. When the end-plate potential has decreased below the threshold necessary to trigger the action potential in the muscle fibre, conduction ceases. Any effective local increase in concentration of acetyl choline, such as may be due to repetitive stimulation of the motor nerve, will antagonise the effect. Competitive block is characteristically antagonised by acetyl choline and by other anticholinesterases.

4. *Depolarisation block* is due to prolonged depolarisation of the motor end-plate. This type of block may be produced by acetyl choline itself in high dosage or by anticholinesterases such as neostigmine, or by substances which mimic the action of acetyl choline by combining with the receptor of ACh to form an active complex and depolarise the post-synaptic membrane. Examples of this type of drug are decamethonium and suxamethonium. In this type of block the end-plate depolarisation is initially associated with excitation or increased excitability, and paralysis may be preceded by fasciculations. The block once present is not easily antagonised, anticholinesterases and previous tetanisation having no effect. Substances which raise the end-plate threshold to acetyl choline, such as curare, may reverse it. There is considerable species difference in the response to acetyl choline-like drugs, and in many mammals, including monkey, dog, and rabbit, there is a dual type of response in which the depolarisation block is followed by a different form of block which is deepened by curare and antagonised by neostigmine, and which may resemble a competitive type of block. This dual response may occur in the human subject in normal neonates.

In myasthenia gravis, while it is clearly established that there is a disturbance in neuromuscular transmission, the site of the block is still uncertain and the possible relevance of electrophysiological studies to this question will be considered below.

THE JOLLY EFFECT

Although it was not established that the defect in myasthenia gravis was one of neuromuscular transmission until 1934, when Mary Walker showed that treatment with physostigmine was effective,

Jolly in 1895 showed clearly that the defect was peripheral in situation. He showed that, if a muscle is stimulated through its motor nerve by applying a faradic current to the muscle, there is an initial brisk contraction followed by a falling off of tension. It was later demonstrated that the tension could be restored by direct stimulation of the muscle by a galvanic current (Campbell and Bramwell, 1900). This sequence of events is known as the myasthenic reaction. Its diagnostic value may be enhanced if it can be shown that it may be influenced by neostigmine, but as a means of studying neuromuscular transmission it has been superseded by the study of evoked potentials following neuromuscular stimulation at different rates.

THE VOLUNTARY ELECTROMYOGRAM

In myasthenia gravis, spontaneous activity is rarely observed in resting muscle when electromyography is performed using a needle electrode. During voluntary contractions, normal motor unit action potentials may be obtained, but during sustained effort in an affected muscle there is a gradual reduction in amplitude of the interference pattern. During the final stage of exhaustion, the interference pattern is lost, and it is possible to record single units which may appear to drop out suddenly. The electrical activity may be rapidly restored by giving the patient an anticholinesterase such as edrophonium.

Although many patients may show motor unit potentials which have an entirely normal appearance, it is not uncommon to see potentials which are abnormally polyphasic and resemble the potentials which are seen in muscular dystrophy. It is likely that several mechanisms are involved here. One is that in severely affected muscle, neuromuscular block may affect some fibres in a unit more than others, so that during a contraction only some of the fibres in the units give rise to action potentials, and the unit as a whole is polyphasic. In longstanding myasthenia certain muscles may develop weakness which does not respond to neostigmine, and this is due to myopathic changes developing in the muscle, and gives rise to the appearance of polyphasic units in the electromyogram. Difficulty may arise from the fact that symptomatic myasthenia may be a feature of polymyositis, and the presence of a marked excess of insertion activity, of fibrillation, and positive saw-tooth potentials, may be valuable in distinguishing this condition from myasthenia gravis (Simpson, 1963).

NEUROMUSCULAR STIMULATION

Neuromuscular block may be studied in patients by recording evoked potentials from a muscle after repetitive stimulation of its nerve. A useful arrangement is to stimulate the ulnar nerve at the wrist or elbow and record evoked potentials through surface electrodes applied over the abductor digiti minimi. If supramaximal stimuli are employed, changes in size of the evoked potential may be used to measure the degree of neuromuscular block. Movement artefact is a major difficulty in this procedure, which can be reduced to some extent by splinting the limb. Although surface electrodes have been most widely used in clinical testing, subcutaneous recording electrodes have been recommended as giving rise to less artefact (Slomić et al., 1968).

A healthy subject will tolerate repetitive stimulation at low rates of frequency for long periods without any decline in the size of the evoked potential. If stimulation is carried out at a rate of more than 10 a second, the first 3 to 5 stimuli are followed by a progressive increase in the amplitude of the evoked potential which becomes shorter in duration. Both these effects may be related to an increase in the synchronisation of the muscle response. At 100 to 200 msec from the start of stimulation there may be an artefact of movement which gives rise to a transient reduction in amplitude. If the muscle is stimulated at tetanic frequency there may be a decline in amplitude of the evoked potentials, which varies between different individuals and with the rate of stimulation. During a period of 3 sec there is no appreciable change in size with frequencies of up to 40 a second. At rates above 65 a second the voltage may fall to half its value in 5 to 10 sec. At 50 a second it may take 30 sec, or longer, for the evoked potential to fall to 50 per cent of the initial value. If tetanic stimulation is interrupted and stimulation at a slow rate is resumed, the potentials usually revert to the value obtaining before the tetanus (Harvey and Masland, 1941; Simpson, 1966).

In myasthenia gravis, the changes vary considerably between different patients and according to the severity of the disease. In some individuals, if a single pair of stimuli is administered separated by anything from 20 msec to 2 sec, the amplitude of the second potential may be significantly less than that of the first. In such a person, repetitive stimulation at as low a rate as 3 a second may be followed by a progressive decline in size of the evoked potentials. On the other hand, this is not an invariable finding, and in some

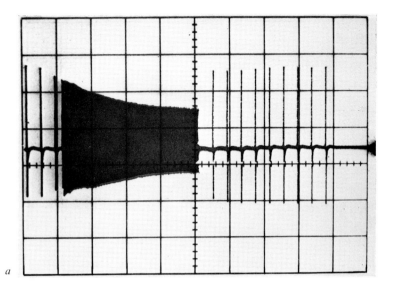

a

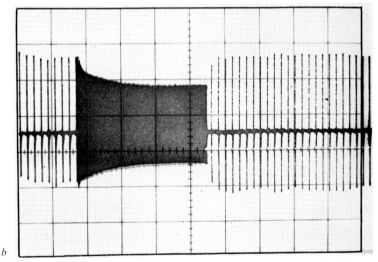

b

PLATE 13 Evoked potentials in patient with myasthenia gravis obtained from abductor digiti minimi following repetitive stimulation of the ulnar nerve. In each record stimulation is at 5 and 50 c/s. Height of squares in graticule represents 2.0 mv. In record (*a*) amplitude of potentials decreases both at 5/sec and at 50/sec. In record (*b*) amplitude of potentials only decreases at 50/sec, but the amplitude is increased following tetanic stimulation.

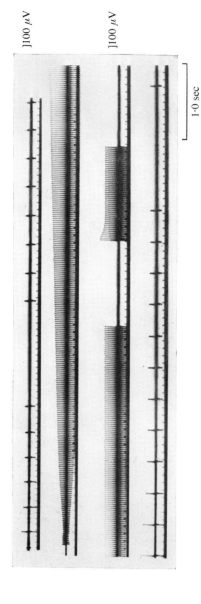

]100 μV

]100 μV

1·0 sec

PLATE 14 Carcinomatous myasthenia. Sub-maximal response with decrement to 2·3 stimuli/sec. Progressive increment at 50/sec. (By courtesy of J. A. Simpson and *Proc. roy. Soc. Med.*)

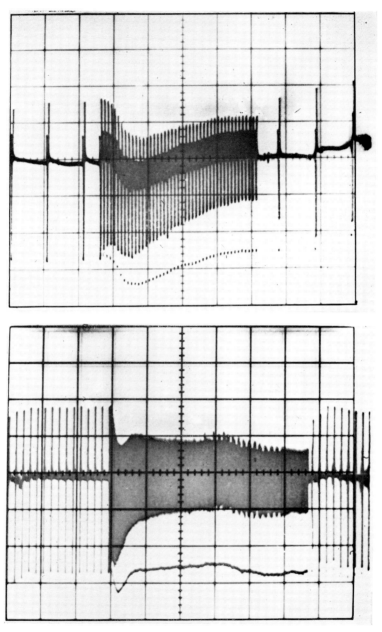

PLATE 15 Fall in amplitude of potentials evoked in abductor digiti minimi during tetanic stimulation of the ulnar nerve in patient with motor neurone disease. In each record stimulation is at 5 and 50 c/s. Height of squares on graticule represents 500 μv.

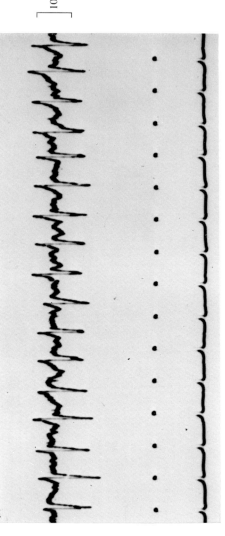

PLATE 16 Reduced motor unit activity in partially denervated lateral rectus muscle of patient with paralytic strabismus. Time scale 10 msec.

100 μV

PLATE 17 (below) Ocular Myopathy. The upper record shows the discharge recorded from the lateral rectus with the eye in the primary position. In the lower record increased activity is recorded during attempted abduction although the eye was not

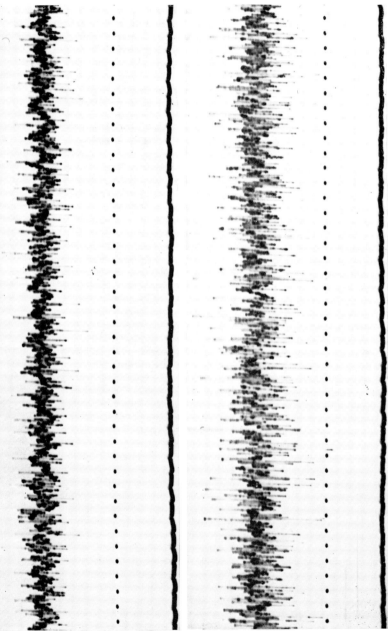

a

b

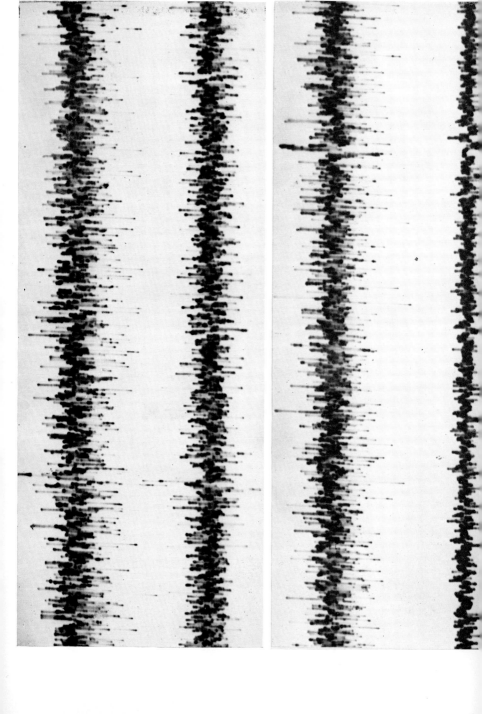

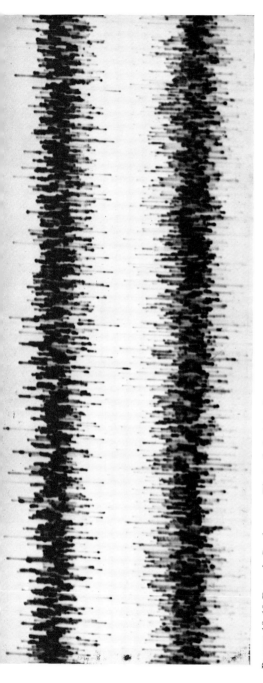

100 msec

PLATES 18, 19 Duane's Syndrome. Electrode in lateral rectus (upper channel) and medial rectus (lower channel). In upper record eye is in primary position and the resting discharge is equal in both muscles. In centre record showing attempted abduction there is activity in the lateral rectus and almost complete inhibition in the medial rectus. In the lower record, which shows attempted adduction, although the medial rectus is discharging strongly there is failure of inhibition of the lateral rectus.

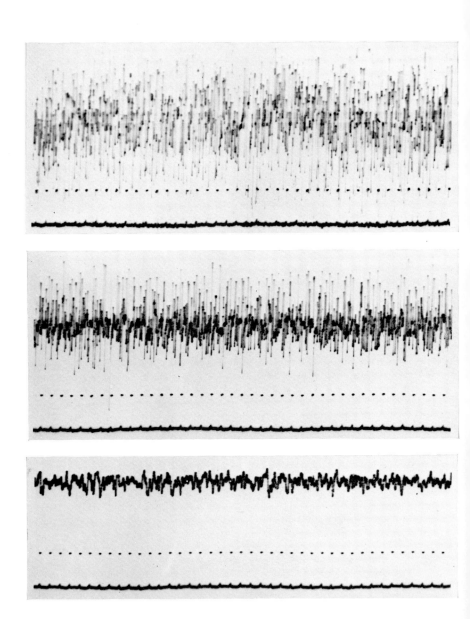

PLATE 20 Myasthenia gravis. Three successive records from the external rectus of a patient with myasthenia gravis showing the decrement in unit activity during sustained contraction. Time scale 10 msec.

individuals there may be no decline in amplitude except with a full tetanus, while in others fatigue may be demonstrated with slow rates of stimulation only when this follows successive bursts of tetanus. The response to a tetanus is likewise variable, but the most characteristic response to a rate of stimulation at 50 a second is for a decrement to occur immediately, or very soon, after the onset of the tetanus and continue for 1 to 2 sec, after which the potential is maintained at a much reduced, but no longer decrementing, level. In some cases there may be little decrement with the first tetanus, but after successive bursts the classical myasthenic response may be obtained. An important type of response which may be seen in myasthenia gravis, although it is more characteristic of symptomatic myasthenias, is for the tetanus to show an incrementing type of response. This is sometimes associated with a decrementing response at slow rates of stimulation (Simpson, 1960, 1966).

Following a tetanus in myasthenia gravis, there is often an increase in the action potential response to single shocks delivered after the termination of the tetanus (Plate 13). This is more pronounced the greater the frequency or duration of the tetanus. It is similar to the post tetanic facilitation which occurs after the administration of curare, and which has been shown to be due to increased output of acetyl choline from the nerve endings following the tetanus (Grob et al., 1956). The post tetanic facilitation occurring in myasthenia gravis differs from that seen after curarisation in that, if stimulation is continued at a slow rate after the tetanus, there is a progressive fall in the size of the action potential over about 20 min. This is very similar to what is seen in animals after the administration of hemicholinium, and has led Desmedt (1958) to argue that the defect in myasthenia is primarily due to failure of release of acetyl choline, rather than to a postsynaptic competitive-type block (see Chapter 3).

EFFECT OF DRUGS ON MYASTHENIC BLOCK

The similarity of the neuromuscular block in myasthenia gravis to that seen following the administration of curare has been referred to above. Curare may be used to confirm the diagnosis of myasthenia, since in myasthenia it may provoke increased weakness in a low dose which has no effect on a healthy subject. Quinine bisulphate, which has a curare-like action may be used for the same purpose, but both these drugs may produce severe weakness in myasthenics and are not without risk.

The most useful pharmacological test is the administration of endrophonium chloride. This has a short duration anticholinesterase action and 10 mg (after an initial test dose of 2 mg) may be given intravenously. If there is clinical weakness, improvement will take place in about 1 min and last about 5 min. Likewise, the electrical fatigue effect on evoked potentials may be abolished during this time. Neostigmine may be used in a similar manner to produce an anti-myasthenic effect, but is less generally useful because of its more prolonged latency and greater duration of action.

The action of decamethonium in myasthenia is of interest, because it differs from that which follows the use of the drug on healthy subjects (Churchill-Davidson and Richardson, 1952). In mildly affected patients, the muscles are much less sensitive to the depolarising action of decamethonium than is healthy muscle. In the more severely affected patients decamethonium will produce neuromuscular block, but the depolarisation block is relatively short-lived and is rapidly succeeded by a competitive-type block, reversible with tensilon or neostigmine. This altered response to drugs is of interest, in view of the species differences in response to decamethonium. Grob *et al.* (1956) have shown that acetyl choline itself has a different effect on myasthenic than normal subjects, in that it also gives rise initially to a fleeting depolarisation followed by a competitive-type block. These findings could all indicate that myasthenic muscle has different membrane characteristics from normal muscle.

SYMPTOMATIC MYASTHENIA
In polymyositis, electrical stimulation of a nerve may be followed by a myasthenic-like response to a tetanus. This is usually a decrementing type of response, but sometimes a progressive increase in the amplitude of the evoked potentials during the tetanus is seen. There is usually little change with slow rates of stimulation, and the response to neostigmine or tensilon is not striking.

A myasthenic syndrome which is similar in some respects to that seen in polymyositis may occur in association with bronchial carcinoma. If the nerve is stimulated at a slow rate (1 to 2 a second), there is a progressive reduction in size of the evoked muscle potentials. On the other hand, with rapid rates of stimulation there is a progressive increase in the size of the potential (Plate 14). Post tetanic facilitation may occur, but is short-lived and is followed by the post tetanic exhaustion described by Desmedt in myasthenia gravis. There is usually a poor response to neostigmine, but in contrast to myasthenia gravis there may be an increased sensitivity to depolarising agents such as decamethonium. Recently, it has been shown that administration of guanidine, which promotes the release of acetyl choline from the nerve endings, produces a clinical improvement and may reverse the electrical abnormality. The incrementing response to tetanic stimulation is similar to that which may be seen in botulinus intoxication, and this together with the effect of guanidine would favour the view that in this syndrome the abnormality involves a defect in acetyl choline release (Rooke et al., 1960; McQuillen and Jons, 1967; Elmqvist and Lambert, 1968) (see also Chapter 3).

NEUROMUSCULAR BLOCK IN LOWER MOTOR NEURONE LESIONS

In 1948, Hodes described fatigue of evoked potentials in patients with lower motor neurone lesions due to poliomyelitis. More recently, a decremental response to tetanic stimulation of a peripheral nerve has been described in motor neurone disease and some forms of peripheral neuropathy (Mulder et al., 1959; Simpson and Lenman, 1959). These changes occur irregularly and are of limited diagnostic value, but may give rise to confusion in that they may enable a diagnosis of myasthenia gravis to be made in error (Plate 15). The response to edrophonium and neostigmine, however, is much less marked than in myasthenia. The underlying mechanism of this phenomenon in lower motor neurone lesions is unknown, but one possibility is that disease affecting the anterior horn cells may interfere either with the synthesis or release of acetyl choline (Simpson, 1966). In motor neurone disease and poliomyelitis, where collateral sprouting of the surviving axons may be prominant, the possibility also exists that chemical transmission may be abnormal across the end-plates of the regenerating sprouts.

12
The Ocular Muscles

The muscles that move the eyball are concerned with rapid accurately controlled movements, and movements of the eye depend on the joint action of groups of muscles acting in association, so that the nervous control is relatively complex. The principle of reciprocal innervation is particularly adapted to the movements of the eye, since these depend on the simultaneous contraction and relaxation of opposing muscles. The capacity of the eye muscles for rapid controlled movement is associated with important characteristics affecting both the structure of the muscles and their mode of innervation. The diameter of the muscle fibres is small, and the innervation ratio is low, so that the motor units contain very few muscle fibres compared to the motor units in the skeletal muscle of the limbs (Buchthal, 1960; Sissons, 1964). The muscle fibres are also activated by nerve impulses firing at more rapid rates than is usual with skeletal muscle elsewhere in the body. These changes are reflected in the electromyogram, which has made a useful contribution to the study of the function and organisation of the extra-ocular muscles.

The clinical application of electromyography to the ocular muscles was first reported by Björk and Kugelberg (1953a), and has been extensively reviewed by Breinin (1962). It gives particularly precise information regarding the synergic action of the different ocular muscles, and this of value in the interpretation of squint. A limitation in this connection is that children do not tolerate the procedure as readily as adults. In the analysis of paralytic squint, it may be useful to identify partial denervation and to distinguish neurogenic weakness from that due to an ocular myopathy, and it may clarify the situation when the action of the eye muscles is affected by trauma or by fascial bands. Whereas the diagnosis of myasthenia gravis is generally made and established by other means, electromyography of the ocular muscles may sometimes provide additional information of clinical value.

TECHNIQUE

The technical requirements for recording potentials from the extra-ocular muscles are similar to those for recording from muscles elsewhere in the body. On account of the small size of the muscles, it is necessary to use electrodes of particularly fine gauge. If unipolar electrodes are employed, it is necessary to have an additional in-different electrode placed elsewhere. In practice, concentric elec-trodes are satisfactory provided they are of 30 s.w.g. or smaller. The examination is normally conducted with the patient lying horizontal and the gaze directed forwards. Before the electrodes are inserted, the eye is anaesthetised with a few drops of topical local anaesthetic. To insert the electrode the conjunctiva over the tendon of the muscle may be picked up with fine forceps, and the electrode passed into the belly of the muscle slightly obliquely to its long axis. Further adjustment of the position of the electrode may be necessary until an interference pattern is recognised on the oscilloscope, or by the loudspeaker monitor. In order to study the interaction of different muscles, it is frequently an advantage to insert a pair of electrodes, each in an antagonist muscle, and this can generally be tolerated by the patient without undue discomfort. Complications of this procedure are uncommon, but, occasionally, subconjunctival ecchymoses may occur (Björk and Kugelberg, 1953a; Marg et al., 1959; Breinin, 1962).

THE NORMAL EXTRA-OCULAR ELECTROMYOGRAM

The pattern of motor unit recruitment in the external ocular muscles is, in many respects, similar to that in muscles elsewhere in the body, but the characteristic structure of the eye muscles and their capacity for rapid movement is associated with distinctive electromyographic features. The motor units contain less than 20 muscle fibres (Torre, 1953), compared to between 100 and 2,000 fibres/unit in the muscles of the limbs (Feinstein et al., 1955), and, consequently, the motor unit potentials are brief and of comparatively low amplitude. Thus, the mean duration of action potentials in the recti has been recorded as 1.60 ± 0.06 msec, and the mean amplitude as $108.0 \pm 9.2\ \mu$V compared with 6.74 ± 0.28 msec, and $394.0 \pm 26.0\ \mu$V in the first dorsal interosseus muscle (Björk and Kugelberg, 1953a). The action potentials are relatively uniform in shape, and are rarely polyphasic. Relatively rapid rates of motor unit firing have been recorded in the extra-ocular muscles. In the muscles of the limbs, rates of firing of greater than 50 a second are unusual, although rates of up to 100 a second have been recorded (Seyffarth, 1941; Bigland and Lippold, 1954; Norris and Gasteiger, 1955). On the other hand, in paretic muscles of the eye, where individual units can be identified, it has been possible to observe the same potential recurring at a rate of 200 a second (Björk and Kugelberg, 1953a).

On insertion of an electrode into the extra-ocular muscle, brief trains of insertion activity may be observed similar to that recorded elsewhere. In the primary position of the eye the extra-ocular muscles are contracting continuously, so that when an electrode is situated in any of the extra-ocular muscles, with the eye in the primary position, continuous electrical activity is recorded. When the eye moves to one or other side, the electrical activity in the muscle bringing about the movement is increased, and that in its antagonist is decreased (see Plates 18 and 19). This relaxation may be incomplete in a slow deviation of the eye, but in a rapid movement contraction of the active muscle may be accompanied by complete relaxation of its antagonist (Björk and Kugelberg, 1953b).

Although electrical activity is always present in the extra-ocular muscles of the waking subjects, except during reciprocal inhibition, there is a falling off in electrical activity during sleep. This is particularly prominent during surgical anaesthesia, when electrical activity gradually diminishes as the depth of anaesthesia is increased. In deep anaesthesia, the eyes assume a position of divergence and all electrical activity ceases. Thus, in anaesthesia it would appear that the eye is devoid of active innervation, and assumes a resting position dependent on its anatomical situation (Breinin, 1957c, 1962).

DISORDERS OF OCULAR MOVEMENT

NEUROGENIC WEAKNESS

Paralytic squint due to lesions affecting the third, fourth, or sixth cranial nerves is common and the electrical signs of neurogenic weakness are characteristic.

Although fibrillation potentials may be recorded from the extra-ocular muscles in the presence of partial denervation, they are relatively difficult to recognise as they closely resemble the small motor unit potentials which arise from these muscles. Moreover, complete relaxation of the eye muscles does not normally occur, except during full contraction of an antagonist muscle, so they will not normally be seen, except in the presence of motor unit activity, unless the muscle is totally paralysed. In practice, they cannot be identified with certainty unless their occurrence can be seen to be unrelated to any voluntary movement of the eye (Björk, 1954). The most characteristic and readily recognised sign of neurogenic paralysis of an eye muscle is reduced motor unit activity on attempted voluntary contraction. In total paralysis the muscle may be electrically silent, apart from fibrillations, or, in less severe lesions, the electrical pattern may be reduced to single unit activity. Frequently, there is markedly impaired recruitment of motor units, and the interference pattern during maximal effort may have an uneven character resulting from the jerking movements of paretic nystagmus. Polyphasic units are not usually seen, probably on account of the small size of the motor units, but sometimes the motor unit potentials in partially denervated muscle are abnormally prolonged and may have a duration of up to 3·0 msec (Plate 16).

In paralytic squint, electromyography is of value in determining precisely which muscles are affected, and in determining the severity of the paresis. It is of assistance in assessing the prognosis, since fibrillation in paralysed muscle implies denervation and, hence, a slow recovery, and the return of motor unit activity to a paralysed muscle may herald subsequent clinical improvement. It is an aid to diagnosis, in that it may distinguish paralytic squint from squint due to various forms of pseudoparesis, such as may arise from traumatic dislocation of the globe, abnormal tendon attachments, or interference with muscle activity by fascial bands. In such conditions, the apparently paralysed muscles may show normal electrical activity. Electromyography may also serve to distinguish paralytic squint due to disordered innervation from squint caused by ocular myopathy, and myasthenia gravis (Björk, 1954; Breinin, 1957b).

OCULAR MYOPATHY

In neurogenic weakness resulting from lesions affecting the lower motor neurone, the electromyographic findings are conditioned by the fact that there is loss of motor units, so that fewer can be recruited during muscular contraction and the interference pattern on maximal effort may be reduced or absent. In weakness due to muscle disease, the number of motor units is not reduced until a late stage, but there is loss of fibres within the units, which may be of abnormally short duration and polyphasic. Because there is no significant reduction in the number of motor units, the interference pattern is preserved, although it may be of reduced amplitude. In an ocular myopathy, the striking feature in a severe case is that the electrical activity may appear almost normal with a good interference pattern, even although the muscle is apparently completely paralysed (Plate 17). Because the motor unit potentials of the eye muscles are normally of short duration, it is difficult for the eye to detect any significant difference between the characteristics of normal and myopathic units in the extra-ocular muscles. Automatic frequency analysis has been employed to try to demonstrate the higher mean frequency of the myopathic interference pattern (Breinin, 1962), but, since the frequency distribution of the interference pattern of normal ocular muscle lies at the upper end of the frequency spectrum, this method is difficult to apply in clinical practice. Therefore, the most useful diagnostic feature in ocular myopathy is the presence of a good interference pattern in an apparently paretic muscle. This finding is of value in confirming the diagnosis in an advanced case of ocular myopathy, but the recognition of early cases by electromyographic means may be difficult.

MYASTHENIA GRAVIS

In myasthenia gravis, weakness or paralysis of the extra-ocular muscles is one of the commoner presentations. The weakness is characteristically one which increases with fatigue, and the degree to which different muscles are affected is characteristically variable. Electromyographic study may show that the amount of motor unit activity during a sustained contraction falls off progressively (Plate 20). The diagnosis may be confirmed by the administration of edrophonium, which may be followed by the rapid return of motor unit activity to normal (Breinin, 1957a). In patients who are under treatment, a clinical deterioration may indicate either a myasthenic block due to an exacerbation of the disease or a cholinergic block due to overmedication. When myasthenia affects one group of muscles predominantly, a myasthenic and a cholinergic block may coexist in the same person, since the dose of neostigmine required to act on the severely affected muscles may cause a cholinergic block in less affected muscles. In a cholinergic block, the administration of edrophonium may result in a further fall off in motor unit activity during attempted muscular contraction. Sometimes, in myasthenia gravis, myopathic changes take place in the affected muscles which become resistant to neostigmine, and this change is not uncommon in the ocular muscles in myasthenia. In such instances, if electromyography is carried out the motor unit activity in the paretic muscles is not enhanced by edrophonium.

CONGENITIAL MUSCULOFASCIAL ANOMALIES
In this group of conditions, there may be partial replacement of certain of the extra-ocular muscles by fibrous tissue, and, in addition, abnormal bands of fascia may connect one muscle with another. The anomalies may affect gaze, either in the vertical or horizontal plane, and, generally, there is limitation of movement of the eye in at least one direction of gaze. When the eye is moved in the opposite direction to that in which movement is limited, retraction of the eyeball may occur.

Electromyographic study of this group of conditions has been limited by the difficulty in applying the procedure to children, but the technique has yielded useful information in Duane's retraction syndrome. In this condition, abduction of the eye is impaired and there may also be some restriction of adduction, which may be associated with ptosis and retraction of the globe. The underlying abnormality is not fully understood, but it has been suggested that retraction may result from the pull of a fibrotic lateral rectus which is unable to relax reciprocally (Breinin, 1957b). The characteristic electromyographic findings are that the lateral rectus may show reduced activity both in the primary position and on attempted abduction. On attempted adduction, the lateral rectus muscle fails to relax (Plates 18 and 19).

Bibliography

Adrian, E. D. (1916) The electrical reactions of muscle before and after injury, *Brain*, **39**, 1–33.

Adrian, E. D. (1917) Physiological basis of electrical tests in peripheral nerve injury, *Arch. Radiol. Electrother.*, **21**, 379–92.

Adrian, E. D. and Bronk, D. W. (1929) The discharge of impulses in motor nerve fibres, *J. Physiol. (Lond.)*, **67**, 119–51.

Adrian, R. H. (1956) Effect of internal and external potassium concentration on the membrane potential of frog muscle, *J. Physiol. (Lond.)*, **133**, 631–58.

Amick, L. D. and Lemmi, H. (1963) Electromyographic studies in peroneal muscular atrophy, *Arch. Neurol. (Chic.)*, **5**, 472–82.

Araki, T. and Otani, T. (1955) Response of single motoneurones to direct stimulation in toad's spinal cord, *J. Neurophysiol.*, **18**, 472–85.

Åstrom- K-E., Kugelberg, E. and Müller, R. (1961) Hypothyroid myopathy, *Arch. Neurol. (Chic.)*, **5**, 472–82.

Axelsson, J. and Thesleff, S. (1959) A study of supersensitivity in denervated mammalian skeletal muscle, *J. Physiol. (Lond.)*, **147**, 177–93.

Baccaredda-Boy, A., Mastropaoli, C., Pastorino, P., Sacco, G. and Farris, G. (1963) Electromyographic findings in leprosy, *Int. J. Leprosy.*, **31**, 531–2.

Barwick, D. D. (1963) Investigation of the carrier state in the Duchenne type dystrophy, in *Research in Muscular Dystrophy*, Proc. 2nd Symp. on Current Res. Muscular Dystrophy, pp. 10–19, London: Pitman Medical.

Basmajian, J. V. (1968) *Muscles Alive: Their Functions Revealed by Electromyography*, 2nd ed., Baltimore: Williams & Wilkins.

Bauwens, P. (1956) Variations of the motor unit, *Proc. roy. Soc. Med.*, **49**, 110–11.

Bauwens, P. and Richardson, A. T. (1950) Electrodiagnosis, in *Recent Advances in Physical Medicine*, Ed. F. Bach, pp. 61–82. London: Churchill.

Belmar, J. and Eyzaguirre, C. (1966) Pacemaker site of fibrillation potentials in denervated mammalian muscle, *J. Neurophysiol.*, **29**, 425–41.

Bernhard, C. G., Granit, R. and Skoglund, C. R. (1942) Breakdown of accommodation; nerve as a model-sense organ, *J. Neurophysiol.*, **5**, 55–68.

Beranek, R. (1964) Intracellular stimulation myography in man, *Electroenceph. clin. Neurophysiol.*, **16**, 301–4.

Berry, C. M., Grundfest, H. and Hinsey, J. C. (1944) The electrical activity of regenerating nerves in the cat, *J. Neurophysiol.*, **7**, 103–15.

Bigland, B. and Lippold, O. C. J. (1954) Motor unit activity in the voluntary contraction of human muscle, *J. Physiol. (Lond.)*, **125**, 322–35.

Bischoff, A. and Esslen, E. (1965) Myopathy with primary hyperparathyroidism, *Neurology (Minneap.)*, **15**, 64–8.

Björk, A. (1954) Electromyographic study of conditions involving limited mobility of the eye, chiefly due to neurogenic pareses, *Brit. J. Ophthal.*, **38**, 528–44.

Björk, A. and Kugelberg, E. (1953a) Motor unit activity in the human extraocular muscles, *Electroenceph. clin. Neurophysiol.*, **5**, 271–8.

Björk, A. and Kugelberg, E. (1953b) The electrical activity of the muscles of the eye and eyelids in various positions and during movement, *Electroenceph. clin. Neurophysiol.*, **5**, 595–602.

Bonney, G. and Gilliatt, R. W. (1958) Sensory nerve conduction after traction lesions of the brachial plexus, *Proc. roy. Soc. Med.*, **51**, 365–7.

Bordet, E. (1907) Le traitement de l'atrophie musculaire par les courants galvaniques ondules, *Arch. Élect. méd.*, **15**, 452–61.

Boyd, I. A. (1964) The morphology of muscle spindles and tendon organs, in *The Role of the Gamma System in Movement and Posture*, by Boyd, I. A., Eyzaguirre, C., Matthews, P. B. C. and Rushworth, G. New York: Association for the Aid of Crippled Children.

Breinin, G. M. (1957a) Electromyography—a tool in ocular and neurologic diagnosis: I. Myasthenia gravis, *Arch. Ophthal.*, **57**, 161–4.

Breinin, G. M. (1957b) Electromyography—a tool in ocular and neurologic diagnosis: II. Muscle Palsies, *Arch. Ophthal.*, **57**, 165–75.

Breinin, G. M. (1957c) The position of rest during anaesthesia and sleep, *Arch. Ophthal.*, **57**, 323–6.

Breinin, G. M. (1962) *The Electrophysiology of Extraocular Muscle.* Toronto: University of Toronto Press.

Brennand, R. (1959) Recommendations for medical electronic instrumentation, *J. Brit. I.R.E.*, **19**, 245–51.

Brown, G. L. (1937) The actions of acetylcholine on denervated mammalian and frog's muscle, *J. Physiol. (London.)*, **89**, 438–61.

Brown, G. L. and Harvey, A. M. (1939) Congenital myotonia in the goat, *Brain*, **62**, 341–63.

Brown, M. C. and Matthews, P. B. C. (1966) On the subdivision of the efferent fibres to muscle spindles into static and dynamic fusimotor units, in *The Control and Innervation of Skeletal Muscle*, Ed. B. L. Andrew. Edinburgh: E. & S. Livingstone.

Bryant, S. H. (1962) Muscle membrane of normal and myotonic goats in normal and low external chloride, *Fed. Proc.*, **21**, 312.

Buchthal, F. (1960) The general concept of the motor unit, in 'Neuromuscular disorders', *Res. Publ. Ass. nerv. ment. Dis.*, **38**, 3–30.

Buchthal, F. (1966) Spontaneous and voluntary electrical activity in neuromuscular disorders, *Bull. N.Y. Acad. Med.*, **42**, 521–50.

Buchthal, F. and Clemmeson, S. (1941) On the differentiation of muscle atrophy by electromyography, *Acta psychiat. (Kbh.)*, **16**, 145–81.

Buchthal, F. and Clemmeson, S. (1943) The electromyogram of atrophic muscles in cases of intramedullary affections, *Acta psychiat. (Kbh.)*, **18**, 377–87.

Buchthal, F. and Engbaek, L. (1963) Refractory period and conduction velocity in striated muscle fibres, *Acta physiol. scand.*, **59**, 199–220.

Buchthal, F., Engbaek, L. and Gamstrop, I. (1958) Paresis and hyperexcitability in adynamia episodica hereditaria, *Neurology (Minneap.)*, **8**, 347–51.

Buchthal, F., Erminio, F. and Rosenfalck, P. (1959) Motor unit territory in different human muscles, *Acta physiol. scand.*, **45**, 72–87.

Buchthal, F., Guld, C. and Rosenfalck, P. (1954) Action potential parameters in normal muscle and their dependence on physical variables, *Acta physiol. scand.*, **32**, 200–18.

Buchthal, F., Guld, C. and Rosenfalck, P. (1955) Propagation velocity in electrically activated muscle fibres in man, *Acta physiol. scand.*, **34**, suppl. 120, 75–89.

Buchthal, F. and Madsen, A. (1950) Synchronous activity in normal and atrophic muscle, *Electroenceph. clin. Neurophysiol.*, **2**, 425–44.

Buchthal, F. and Pinelli, P. (1952) Analysis of muscle action potentials as a diagnostic aid in neuromuscular disorders, *Acta med. scand.*, **142**, suppl. 226, 315–27.

Buchthal, F. and Pinelli, P. (1953) Muscle action potentials in polymyositis, *Neurology (Minneap.)*, **3**, 424–36.

Buchthal, F. and Pinelli, P. (1953) Action potentials in muscular atrophy of neurogenic origin, *Neurology (Minneap.)*, **3**, 591–603.

Buchthal, F., Pinelli, P. and Rosenfalck, P. (1954) Action potential parameters in normal human muscle and their physiological determinants, *Acta physiol. scand.*, **32**, 219–29.

Buchthal, F. and Rosenfalck, A. (1965) Action potentials from sensory nerve in man: physiology and clinical application, *Acta neurol. scand.*, **41**, suppl. 13, 263–6.

Buchthal, F. and Rosenfalck, A. (1966) Evoked action potentials and conduction velocity in human sensory nerves, *Brain Res.*, **3**, 1–122.

Buchthal, F. and Rosenfalck, P. (1963) Electrophysiological aspects of myopathy with particular reference to progressive muscular dystrophy, in *Muscular Dystrophy in Man and Animals*, Eds. G. H. Bourne and M. N. Golarz. Basel: S. Karger.

Buchthal, F. and Rosenfalck, P. (1966) Spontaneous electrical activity of human muscle *Electroenceph. clin. Neurophysiol.*, **20**, 321–36.

Buchthal, F., Rosenfalck, P. and Erminio, F. (1960) Motor unit territory and fiber density in myopathies, *Neurology (Minneap.)*, **10**, 398–408.

Buller, A. J., Eccles, J. C. and Eccles, Rosamund, M. (1960) Interactions between motoneurones and muscles in respect of the characteristic speeds of their responses. *J. Physiol. (Lond.)*, **150**, 417–39.

Campbell, H. and Bramwell, E. (1900) Myasthenia gravis, *Brain*, **23**, 277–336.

Caruso, G. and Buchthal, F. (1965) Refractory period of muscle and electromyographic findings in relatives of patients with muscular dystrophy, *Brain*, **88**, 29–50.

Castillo, J. del and Katz, B. (1956) Biophysical aspects of neuromuscular transmission, *Progr. Biophys. molec. Biol.*, **6**, 122–70.

Chopra, J. S. and Hurwitz, L. J. (1968) Femoral conduction in diabetes and chronic occlusive vascular disease, *J. Neurol. Neurosurg. Psychiat.*, **31**, 28–33.

Churchill-Davidson, H. C. and Richardson, A. T. (1952) Action of decamethonium iodide (C 10) in myasthenia gravis, *J. Neurol. Neurosurg. Psychiat.*, **15**, 129–33.

Cluzet, J. J. (1913) Electrodiagnostic au moyen d'un condensateur reglable, *C.R. Soc. Biol. (Paris)*, **74**, 1327–9.

Coërs, C. and Woolf, A. L. (1959) *The Innervation of Muscle, a Biopsy Study.* Oxford: Blackwell.

Copland, J. G. and Davies, C. T. M. (1964) A simple clinical skin electrode, *Lancet*, **i**, 416.

Cragg, B. G. and Thomas, P. K. (1964) Changes in nerve conduction in experimental allergic neuritis, *J. Neurol. Neurosurg. Psychiat.*, **27**, 106–15.

Creutzfeldt, O. D., Abbott, B. C., Fowler, W. M. and Pearson, C. M. (1963) Muscle membrane potentials in episodic adynamia, *Electroenceph. clin. Neurophysiol.*, **15**, 508–19.

Dahlbäck, O., Elmqvist, D., Johns, T. R., Radner, S. and Thesleff, S. (1961) Electrophysiologic study of neuromuscular function in myasthenia gravis, *J. Physiol. (Lond.)*, **156**, 336–43.

Dawson, G. D. (1956) The relative excitability and conduction velocity of sensory and motor nerve fibres in man, *J. Physiol. (Lond.)*, **131**, 436–51.

Dawson, G. D. and Scott, J. W. (1949) The recording of nerve action potentials through skin in man, *J. Neurol. Neurosurg. Psychiat.*, **12**, 259–67.

Denny-Brown D. (1949) The interpretation of the electromyogram, *Arch. Neurol. Psychiat. (Chic.)*, **61**, 99–128.

Denny-Brown, D. (1960) Experimental studies pertaining to hypertrophy, regeneration and degeneration, *Res. Publ. Ass. nerv. ment. Dis.*, **38**, 147–96.

Denny-Brown, D. and Bremner, C. (1944) The effect of percussion of nerve, *J. Neurol. Psychiat.*, **7**, 76–95.

Denny-Brown, D. and Pennybacker, J. B. (1938) Fibrillation and fasciculation in voluntary muscle, *Brain*, **61**, 311–44.

Desmedt, J. E. (1950) Etude experimentale de la degenerascence wallerienne et de la reinnervation du muscle squelettique. Premiere partie; Evolution de la constante de temps d'excitation. Deuxieme partie: Evolution de la constante de temps d'accommodation. *Arch. int. Physiol.*, **58**, 23–68, 125–56.

Desmedt, J. E. (1958) Myasthenic-like features of neuromuscular transmission after administration of an inhibitor of acetyl choline synthesis, *Nature*, **182**, 1673–4.

Diamantopoulos, E. and Olsen, P. Z. (1967) Excitability of motor neurones in spinal shock in man, *J. Neurol. Neurosurg. Psychiat.*, **30**, 427–31.

Donaldson, P. E. K. (1958) *Electronic Apparatus for Biological Research.* London: Butterworth.

Doupe, J. (1943) Studies in denervation: I. The contractility and excitability of denervated muscle, *J. Neurol. Psychiat.*, **6**, 141–53.

Dowling, M. H., Fitch, P. and Willison, R. G. (1968) A special purpose digital computer (Biomac 500) used in the analysis of the human electromyogram, *Electroenceph. clin. Neurophysiol.*, **25**, 570–3.

Downie, A. W. (1964) Studies in nerve conduction, in *Disorders of Voluntary Muscle*, Ed. J. N. Walton. London: Churchill.

Downie, A. W. and Newell, D. J. (1961) Sensory nerve conduction in patients with diabetes mellitus and controls, *Neurology (Minneap.)*, **11**, 876–82.

Downie, A. W. and Scott, T. R. (1967) An improved technique for radial nerve conduction studies, *J. Neurol. Neurosurg. Psychiat.*, **30**, 332–6.

Drager, G. A., Hammill, J. F. and Shy, G. M. (1958) Paramyotonia congenita, *Arch. Neurol. Psychiat. (Chic.)*, **80**, 1–9.

Dyck, P. J. and Lambert, E. H. (1968) Lower motor and primary sensory neuron diseases with peroneal muscular atrophy, *Arch. Neurol. (Chic.)*, **18**, 603–25.

Ebeling, P., Gilliatt, R. W. and Thomas, P. K. (1960) A clinical and electrical study of ulnar nerve lesions in the hand, *J. Neurol. Neurosurg. Psychiat.*, **23**, 1–9.

Edwards, R. G. and Lippold, O. C. J. (1956) The relation between force and integrated electrical activity in fatigued muscle, *J. Physiol. (Lond.)*, **132**, 677–81.

Ekstedt, J. (1964) Human single muscle fibre action potentials, *Acta physiol. scand.*, **61**, suppl. 226, 1–91.

Eldred, E., Granit, R. and Merton, P. A. (1953) Supraspinal control of the muscle spindles and its significance, *J. Physiol. (Lond.)*, **122**, 498–523.

Elmqvist, D., Hofmann, W. W., Kugelberg, J. and Quastel, D. M. J. (1964) An electrophysiological investigation of neuromuscular transmission in myasthenia gravis, *J. Physiol. (Lond.)*, **174**, 417–34.

Elmqvist, D. and Lambert, E. H. (1968) Detailed analysis of neuromuscular transmission in a patient with the myasthenic syndrome associated with bronchogenic carcinoma, *Mayo Clin. Proc.*, **43**, 689–713.

Engel, A. G. (1961) Thyroid function and periodic paralysis, *Amer. J. Med.*, **30**, 327–33.

Erb, W. (1868) Zur Casuistik der Nerven—und Muskelkrankheiten, *Dtsch. Arch. klin. Med.*, **4**, 535–78.

Erb, W. (1869) Zur Pathologie und pathologischr Anatomie periphischer Paralysen, *Dtsch. Arch. klin. Med.*, **5**, 42–93.

Erb, W. (1883) *Handbook of Electro-therapeutics*, translated by L. Putztal, MD. New York: William Wood.

Erminio, P., Buchthal, F. and Rosenfalck, P. (1959) Motor unit territory and muscle fibre concentration in paresis due to peripheral nerve injury and anterior horn cell involvement, *Neurology Minneap.)*, **9**, 657–71.

Farmer, T. W., Buchthal, F. and Rosenfalck, P. (1959) Refractory and irresponsive periods of muscle in progressive muscular dystrophy and paresis due to lower motor neuron involvement, *Neurology (Minneap.)*, **9**, 747–56.

Farmer, T. W., Buchthal, F. and Rosenfalck, P. (1960) Refractory period of human muscle after the passage of a propagated action potential, *Electroenceph. clin. Neurophysiol.*, **12**, 455–66.

Feinstein, B., Lindegard, B., Nyman, E. and Wohlfart, G. (1955) Morphologic studies of motor units in normal human muscles, *Acta anat. (Basel)*, **23**, 127–42.

Fullerton, P. M. (1964) Peripheral nerve conduction in metachromatic leucodystrophy (sulphatide lipidosis), *J. Neurol. Neurosurg. Psychiat.*, **27**, 100–5.

Fullerton, P. M. (1969) Toxic chemicals and peripheral neuropathy: Clinical and epidemiological features, *Proc. roy. Soc. Med.*, **62**, 201–4.

Fullerton, P. M. and Gilliatt, R. W. (1965) Axon reflexes in human motor nerve fibres, *J. Neurol. Neurosurg. Psychiat.* **28**, 1–11.

Gamstorp, I. (1956) Adynamia episodica hereditaria, *Acta paediat.* (*Uppsala*), Suppl. 108, **45**, 1–126.

Gamstorp, I. (1962) A study of transient muscular weakness. *Acta neurol. scand.*, **38**, 3–19.

Gardner-Medwin, D. (1968) Studies of the carrier state in the Duchenne type of muscular dystrophy. 2. Quantitative electromyography as a method of carrier detection, *J. Neurol. Neurosurg. Psychiat.*, **31**, 124–34.

Gassel, M. M. (1963) A study of femoral nerve conduction time, *Arch. Neurol.* (*Chic.*), **9**, 607–14.

Gassel, M. M. (1964) A test of nerve conduction to muscles of the shoulder girdle as an aid in the diagnosis of proximal neurogenic and muscular disease, *J. Neurol. Neurosurg. Psychiat.*, **27**, 200–5.

Gassel, M. M. and Diamantopoules, E. (1964) Pattern of conduction time in the distribution of the radial nerve, *Neurology* (*Minneap.*), **14**, 222–31.

Gassel, M. M. and Trojaborg, W. (1964) Clinical and electrophysiological study of the pattern of conduction times in the distribution of the sciatic nerve, *J. Neurol. Neurosurg. Psychiat.*, **27**, 351–7.

Geschwind, N. A. and Simpson, J. A. (1955) Procaine amide in the treatment of myotonia, *Brain*, **78**, 81–91.

Gilliatt, R. W. (1961) Nerve conduction: motor and sensory, in *Electrodiagnosis and Electromyography*. Ed. Sidney Licht. New Haven, Conn: Elizabeth Licht.

Gilliatt, R. W. (1966) Nerve conduction in human and experimental neuropathies, *Proc. roy. Soc. Med.*, **59**, 989–93.

Gilliatt, R. W., Goodman, H. V. and Willison, R. G. (1961) The recording of lateral popliteal nerve action potentials in man, *J. Neurol. Neurosurg. Psychiat.*, **24**, 305–18.

Gilliatt, R. W. and Sears, T. A. (1958) Sensory nerve action potentials in patients with peripheral nerve lesions, *J. Neurol. Neurosurg. Psychiat.*, **21**, 109–18.

Gilliatt, R. W. and Taylor, J. C. (1959) Electrical changes following section of the facial nerve, *Proc. roy. Soc. Med.*, **52**, 1080–3.

Gilliatt, R. W. and Thomas, P. K. (1960) Changes in nerve conduction with ulnar lesions at the elbow, *J. Neurol. Neurosurg. Psychiat.*, **23**, 312–20.

Gilliatt, R. W. and Willison, R. G. (1962) Peripheral nerve conduction in diabetic neuropathy, *J. Neurol. Neurosurg. Psychiat.*, **25**, 11–8.

Giovine, G. P. (1957) Considerations sur L'utilisation des courbes intensite/temps en electrodiagnostic, *J. Radiol. Electrol.*, **38**, 418–25.

Goodman, H. V. and Gilliatt, R. W. (1961) The effect of treatment on median nerve conduction in patients with carpal tunnel syndrome, *Ann. phys. Med.*, **6**, 137–55.

Graham, J. and Gerard, R. W. (1946) Membrane potentials and excitation of impaled single muscle fibres, *J. cell. comp. physiol.*, **28**, 99–117.

Granger, C. V. (1966) Nerve conduction and correlative clinical studies in a patient with tuberculoid leprosy, *Amer. J. Phys. Med.*, **45**, 244–50.

Greenbaum, D. (1964) Observations on the homogeneous nature and on the pathogenesis of diabetic neuropathy, *Brain*, **87**, 215–32.

Greenbaum, D. and Richardson, P. C., Salmon, M. V. and Urich, H. (1964) Pathological observations on six cases of diabetic neuropathy, *Brain*, **87**, 201–14.

Grob, D., Johns, R. J. and Harvey, A. M. (1956) Studies in neuromuscular function, *Bull. Johns Hopk. Hosp.*, **99**, 115–238.

Grodins, F. S., Osborne, S. L., Johnson, F. R. and Ivy, A. C. (1944) Stimulation of denervated skeletal muscle with alternating current, *Amer. J. Physiol.*, **142**, 216–21.

Grodins, F. S., Osborne, S. L., Johnson, F. R., Arana, S. and Ivy, A. C. (1944) The effect of appropriate electrical stimulation on atrophy of denervated muscle in rat, *Amer. J. Physiol.*, **142**, 222–30.

Guld, C. (1960) *Use of Screened Power Transformers and Output Transformers to Reduce Stimulus Artefact*, Proc. 2nd Internat. Cong. med. Elect. Paris, pp. 25–7. London: Iliffe.

Guld, C. (1961) *The Reduction of Stimulus Interference in Electrophysiology*, Proc. 3rd Internat. Conf. med. Elect. London. Instit. Elect. Eng., pp. 103–105. London: Iliffe.

Haase, G. R. and Shy, G. M. (1960) Pathological changes in muscle biopsies from patients with peroneal muscular atrophy. *Brain*, **83**, 631–7.

Harvey, A. M. and Masland, R. L. (1941) A method for the study of neuromuscular transmission in human subjects, *Bull. Johns Hopk. Hosp.*, **68**, 81–93.

Havard, C. W. H., Campbell, E. D. R., Ross, H. B. and Spence,

A. W. (1963) Electromyographic and histological findings in the muscles of patients with thyrotoxicosis, *Quart. J. Med.*, **32**, 145–63.

Heather, A. J. and Apostolico, M. A. (1959) A reaction of degeneration scanner, *Arch phys. Med.*, **40**, 343–6.

Hed, R., Kirstein, L. and Lundmark, C. (1958) Thyrotoxic myopathy, *J. Neurol. Neurosurg Psychiat.*, **21**, 270–8.

Helmholtz, H. von (1850) Messungen über den zeitlichen Verlauf der Zuckung animalischer Muskeln und die Fortpflanzungsgeschwindigkeit der Reizung in den Nerven, *Joh. Müller's Arch. Anat. Physiol.*, 276–364.

Hill, A. V. (1936) Excitation and Accommodation in Nerve, *Proc. roy. Soc. B*, **119**, 305–55.

Hill, A. V., Katz, B. and Solandt, D. Y. (1936) Nerve excitation by alternating current, *Proc. roy. Soc. B*, **121**, 74–133.

Hnik, P. and Skorpil, V. (1962) Fibrillation activity in denervated muscle, in *The Denervated Muscle*, Ed. E. Gutmann. Prague: Czech Acad. Sci.

Hodes, R. (1948) Electromyographic study of neuromuscular transmission in human poliomyelitis, *Arch. Neurol. Psychiat. (Chic.)*, **60**, 457–73.

Hodes, R. (1949) Selective destruction of large motoneurones by poliomyelitis virus: 1. Conduction velocity of motor nerve fibres of chronic poliomyelitis patients, *J. Neurophysiol.*, **12**, 257–66.

Hodes, R., Larrabee, M. G. and German, W. (1948) The human electromyogram in response to nerve stimulation and the conduction velocity of motor axons, *Arch. Neurol. Psychiat. (Chic.)*, **60**, 340–65.

Hodgkin, A. L. and Horowicz, P. (1959) The influence of potassium and chloride ions on the membrane potential of single muscle fibres, *J. Physiol. (Lond.)*, **148**, 127–260.

Hoffmann, P. (1918) Uber die Beziehungen der Sehnenreflexe zur willkürlichen Bewegung und zum Tonus, *Z. Biol.*, **68**, 351–70.

Hofmann, W. W., Alston, W. and Rowe, G. (1966) A study of individual neuromuscular junctions in myotonia. *Electroenceph. clin. Neurophysiol.*, **21**, 521–37.

Hofmann, W. W., Kundin, J. E. and Farrell, D. F. (1967) The pseudomyasthenic syndrome of Eaton and Lambert: an electrophysiological investigation of neuromuscular transmission in myasthenia gravis. *J. Physiol. (Lond.)*, **174**, 417–34.

Horvath, B. and Proctor, J. B. (1960) Muscular dystrophy. Quantitative studies on the composition of dystrophic muscle, *Res. Publ. Ass. nerv. ment. Dis.*, **38**, 740–66.

Huxley, A. F. (1964) The links between excitation and contraction, *Proc. roy. Soc. B*, **160**, 486–8.

Huxley, A. F. and Niedergerke, R. (1954) Structural changes in muscle during contraction. Interference microscopy of living muscle fibres, *Nature*, **173**, 971–3.

Huxley, H. E. and Hanson, J. (1954) Changes in the cross-striations of muscle during contraction and stretch and their structural interpretation, *Nature*, **173**, 973–5.

Jasper, H. and Ballem, G. (1949) Unipolar electromyograms of normal and denervated human muscle, *J. Neurophysiol.*, **12**, 231–43.

Johns, R. J. (1964) Potential changes in the normal and diseased muscle cell, in *Disorders of Voluntary Muscle*. Ed. J. N. Walton, London: Churchill.

Johnson, E. W., Guyton, J. D. and Olsen, K. J. (1960) Motor nerve conduction velocity studies in poliomyelitis, *Arch. Phys. Med. and Rehab*, **41**, 185–90.

Johnson, E. W. and Olsen, K. J. (1960) Clinical value of motor nerve conduction velocity determination, *J. Amer. med. Ass.*, **172**, 2030–5.

Jolly, F. (1895) Uber myasthenia gravis pseudoparalytica, *Berl. Klin. Wschr.*, 33–4.

Jones, H., Lewis (1913) The use of condenser discharges in electrical testing, *Proc. roy. Soc. Med.*, **6**, 49–61.

Jones, R. V., Lambert, E. H. and Sayre, G. P. (1955) Source of a type of 'insertion activity' in electromyography with evaluation of a histological method of localization, *Arch. phys. Med.*, **36**, 301–10.

Joseph, J. (1960) *Man's Posture, Electromyographic Studies*. Springfield, Illinois: Ch. Thomas.

Kay, R. H. (1966) *Experimental Biology*. London: Chapman and Hall (Science Paperbacks).

Kennard, D. W. (1958) Glass microcapillary electrodes used for measuring potential in living tissues, in *Electronic Apparatus for Biological Research*, by P. E. K. Donaldson. London: Butterworth.

Kleeman, F. J., Partridge, L. D. and Glaser, G. H. (1961) Resting potential and muscle fibre size in hereditary mouse muscle dystrophy, *Amer. J. phys. Med.*, **40**, 219–24.

Kopell, H. P. and Thomson, W. A. L. (1963) Peripheral Entrapment Neuropathies. Baltimore: Williams and Wilkins.

Kugelberg, E. (1944) Accommodation in human nerves, *Acta physiol. scand.*, **8**, Suppl., 24.

Kugelberg, E. (1946) 'Injury activity' and 'trigger zones' in human nerves, *Brain*, **69**, 310–24.

Kugelberg, E. (1947) Electromyograms in muscular disorders, *J. Neurol. Neurosurg. Psychiat.*, **21**, 270–8.

Kugelberg, E. (1949) Electromyography in muscular disorders, *J. Neurol. Neurosurg. Psychiat.*, **12**, 129–36.

Kugelberg, E. and Petersen, I. (1949) 'Insertion activity' in electromyography, *J. Neurol. Neurosurg. Psychiat.*, **12**, 268–73.

Kugelberg, E. and Welander, L. (1956) Heredofamilial juvenile muscular atrophy stimulating muscular dystrophy, *Arch. Neurol. Psychiat.*, **75**, 500–9.

Lambert, E. H. (1962) Diagnostic value of electrical stimulation of motor nerves, *Electroenceph. clin. Neurophysiol.*, Suppl. **22**, 9–19.

Lambert, E. H. and Mulder, D. W. (1963) Nerve conduction in the Guillain-Barré syndrome, *Abstract Int. EMG Meeting Copenhagen*, 16–17.

Lambert, E. H., Underdahl, L. O., Beckett, S. and Mederos, L. O. (1951) A study of the ankle jerk in myxoedema, *J. Clin. Endocrinol.*, **11**, 1186–205.

Landau, W. M. (1951) Synchronisation of potentials and response to direct current stimulation in denervated mammalian muscle, *Electroenceph. clin. Neurophysiol.*, **3**, 169–82.

Landau, W. M. (1952) The essential mechanism in myotonia, *Neurology (Minneap.)*, **2**, 369–88.

Landau, W. M. (1953) Duration of neuromuscular function after nerve section in man, *J. Neurosurg.*, **10**, 64–8.

Langworth, E. P. and Taverner, D. (1963) The prognosis in facial palsy, *Brain*, **86**, 465–80.

Lapicque, L. (1926) *L'excitabilite en Fonction du Temps.* Paris: Press Universitaires de France.

Lawrence, D. G. and Locke, S. (1961) Motor nerve conduction velocity in diabetes, *Arch. Neurol. (Chic.)*, **5**, 483–9.

Lenman, J. A. R. (1959) Quantitative electromyographic changes associated with muscular weakness, *J. Neurol. Neurosurg. Psychiat.*, **22**, 306–10.

Lenman, J. A. R. (1963) Micro-electrode studies in muscle disease, in *Research in Muscular Dystrophy*, Proc. 2nd Symposium, pp. 230–9. London: Pitman Medical.

Lenman, J. A. R. (1965) Effect of denervation on the resting membrane potential of healthy and dystrophic muscle. *J. Neurol. Neurosurg. Psychiat.*, **28**, 525–8.

Lenman, J. A. R. (1966) Quantitative aspects of electromyography, in *Control and Innervation of Skeletal Muscle*. Ed. B. L. Andrew, Edinburgh: Livingstone.

Lenman, J. A. R. (1968) The clinical uses of the electromyogram and nerve conduction velocities, in *Some Aspects of Neurology*. Ed. R. F. Robertson, pp. 132–8. Edinburgh: Roy. Coll. Phys. Edin.

Lenman, J. A. R. (1969) The integration and analysis of the electromyogram and related techniques, in *Disorders of Voluntary Muscle*. Ed. J. N. Walton, 2nd ed. London: Churchill.

Lenman, J. A. R. (1969) Unpublished observations.

Lenman, J. A. R. and Potter, J. L. (1966) Electromyographic measurement of fatigue in rheumatoid arthritis and neuromuscular disease, *Ann. rheum. Dis.*, **25**, 75–84.

Liberson, W. T. (1934) Quelques observations sur l'excitabilite des nerfs et des muscles de l'homme par des courants lentement croissants, *Compt. Rend. Soc. Biol.*, **116**, 1319–22.

Liberson, W. T. (1961) Progressive and alternating currents, in *Electrodiagnosis and Electromyography*. Ed. S. Licht, Connecticut: Licht.

Licht, Sidney (1961) History of electrodiagnosis, in *Electrodiagnosis and Electromyography*. Ed. S. Licht, Connecticut: Licht.

Ling, G. and Gerard, R. W. (1949) The normal membrane potential of frog sartorius muscles, *J. cell. comp. physiol.*, **34**, 383–95.

Lippold, O. C. J. (1952) The relation between integrated action potentials in a human muscle and its isometric tension, *J. Physiol. (Lond.)*, **117**, 492–9.

Lorente De Nó, R. (1947) *Studies from the Rockefeller Inst. for Med. Res.*, 132 (2), Chap. 16, pp. 384–477.

Lucas, K. (1907) On the rate of variation of the exciting current as a factor in electric excitation, *J. Physiol. (Lond.)*, **36**, 253–74.

Lucas, K. (1910) On the refractory period of muscle and nerve, *J. Physiol. (Lond.)*, **39**, 331–40.

Ludin, H. P. (1968) Microelectrode study of normal and dystrophic human muscle, *Electroenceph. Clin. Neurophysiol.*, **25**, 411.

Lüllmann, H. and Pracht, W. (1957) Uber den Einfluss von Acetylcholin auf das Membranpotential denervierter Rattenzwerchfelle, *Experientia (Basel)*, **13**, 288–9.

McArdle, B. (1951) Myopathy due to a defect in glycogen breakdown, *Clin. Sci.*, **10**, 13–35.

McComas, A. J. and Mossawy, S. J. (1964) Muscle fibre resting potentials in normal and dystrophic mice, *Electroenceph. clin. Neurophysiol.*, **17**, 705.

McComas, A. J. and Mrozek, K. (1968) The electrical properties of muscle fibre membranes in dystrophia myotonica and myotonia congenita, *J. Neurol. Neurosurg. Psychiat.*, **31**, 441–7.

McComas, A. J., Mrozek, K. and Bradley, W. G. (1968) The nature of the electrophysiological disorder in adynamia episodica, *J. Neurol. Neurosurg. Psychiat.*, **31**, 448–52.

McKenzie, I. G. (1949) Electrical reactions of muscle in poliomyelitis, *Proc. roy. Soc. Med.*, **42**, 488–90.

McLeod, J. G. and Wray, S. H. (1966) An experimental study of the F wave in the baboon, *J. Neurol. Neurosurg. Psychiat.*, **29**, 196–200.

McQuillen, M. P. and Johns, R. J. (1967) The nature of the defect in the Lambert Eaton Syndrome, *Neurology (Minneap.)*, **17**, 527–36.

Magladery, J. W. and McDougall, D. B. (1950) Electrophysiological studies of nerve and reflex activity in normal man, *Bull. Johns Hopk. Hosp.*, **86**, 265–90.

Magladery, J. W., Porter, W. E., Park, A. M. and Teasdall, R. D. (1951) Electrophysiological studies of nerve and reflex activity in normal man, *Bull. Johns Hopk. Hosp.*, **88**, 499–519.

Magladery, J. W., Teasdall, R. D., Park, A. M. and Languth, H. W. (1952) Electrophysiological studies of reflex activity in patients with lesions of the nervous system, *Bull. Johns Hopk. Hosp.*, **91**, 219–75.

Marg, E., Jampolsky, A. and Tamler, E. (1959) Elements of human extraocular electromyography, *Arch. Ophth.*, **61**, 258–73.

Marinacci, A. A. (1964) Comparative value of measurement of nerve conduction velocity and electromyography in the diagnosis of the carpal tunnel syndrome, *Arch. Phys. Med.*, **45**, 548–54.

Mawdsley, C. and Mayer, R. F. (1965) Nerve conduction in alcoholic polyneuropathy, *Brain*, **88**, 335–56.

Medical Research Council Sub-Committee Report (1958) Electrodiagnostic stimulators, *Brit. med. J.*, **ii**, 714–8.

Medical Research Council War Memorandum No. 7 (1942) *Aids to the Investigation of Peripheral Nerve Injuries.* London: HMSO.

Mulder, D., Calverley, J. R. and Miller, R. (1960) Autogenous Mononeuropathy: diagnosis, treatment and significance, *Med. Clin. N. Amer.*, **44**, 989–99.

Mulder, D. W., Lambert, E. H. and Bastron, J. A. and Sprague, R. G. (1961) The neuropathies associated with diabetes mellitus. A clinical and electromyographic study of 103 unselected diabetic patients, *Neurology (Mineap.)*, **11**, 275–84.

Mulder, D. W., Lambert, E. H. and Eaton, L. M. (1959) Myasthenic syndrome in patients with amyotrophic lateral sclerosis, *Neurology (Minneap.)*, **9**, 627–31.

Myrianthopoulos, N. C., Lane, M. H., Silberberg, D. H. and Vincent, B. L. (1964) Nerve conduction and other studies in families with Charcot-Marie-Tooth disease, *Brain*, **87**, 589–608.

Neilson, J. M. M. (1962) An investigation of methods of recording the electrical activity of the nervous system with particular reference to the occurrence and suppression of stimulus artefact. PhD Thesis University of Edinburgh, 1962.

Newman, H. W. and Livingstone, W. K. (1947) Electrical aids in prognosis of nerve injuries, *J. Neurol. Neurosurg. Psychiat.*, **10**, 118–21.

Nicholls, J. G. (1956) The electrical properties of denervated skeletal muscle, *J. Physiol. (Lond.)*, **131**, 1–12.

Norris, Jr., F. H. (1962) Unstable membrane potential in human myotonic muscle, *Electroenceph. clin. Neurophysiol.*, **14**, 197–201.

Norris, F. H. Jr. and Chatfield, P. O. (1955) Some electrophysiological aspects of muscular dystrophy, *Electroenceph. clin. Neurophysiol.*, **7**, 391–7.

Norris, F. H. and Gasteiger, E. L. (1955) Action potentials of single motor units in normal muscle, *Electroenceph. clin. Neurophysiol.*, **7**, 115–26.

Olsen, P. Z. and Diamantopoulos, E. (1967) Excitability of spinal motor neurones in normal subjects and patients with spasticity, Parkinsonian rigidity and cerebellar hypotonia, *J. Neurol. Neurosurg. Psychiat.*, **30**, 325–31.

Osborne, S. L., Grodins, F. S., Mittelman, E. E., Milne, W. S. and Ivy, A. C. (1944) Rationals for electrodiagnosis and electrical stimulation in denervated muscle, *Arch. phys. Ther.*, **25**, 338–44.

Paillard, J. (1955) Analyse electrophysiologique et comparaison, chez l'homme, du reflexe de Hoffmann et du reflexe myotatique, *Pflügers Archiv.*, **260**, 448–79.

Pearson, C. M., Coleman, R. W., Fowler, W. M., Mommaerts, W. F. H. M., Munsat, T. L. and Peter, J. B. (1967) Skeletal Muscle. Basic and clinical aspects and illustrative new diseases, *Ann. Int. Med.*, **67**, 614–50.

Peiris, O. A. and Miles, D. W. (1965) Galvanic stimulation of the tongue as a prognostic index in Bell's palsy, *Brit. med. J.*, **ii**, 1162–3.

Pinelli, P. and Buchthal, F. (1951) Duration, amplitude and shape of muscle action potentials in poliomyelitis, *Electroenceph. clin. Neurophysiol.*, **3**, 497–504.

Pinelli, P. and Buchthal, F. (1953) Muscle action potentials in myopathies with special regard to progressive muscular dystrophy, *Neurology (Minneap.)*, **3**, 347–59.

Piper, H. (1908) Uber die Leitungsgeschwindigkeit in den markhaltigen, menschlichen Nerven, *Pflügers Arch. ges. Physiol.*, **124**, 591–600.

Piper, H. (1912) *Electrophysiologie Menschlicher Muskeln*. Berlin: Julius Springer.

Pollock, L. J. (1944) Physical therapy and science, *Physiotherapy Rev.*, **24**, 187–9.

Pollock, L. J., Golseth, J. G. and Arieff, A. J. (1945) Galvanic tetanus and galvanic tetanus ratio in electrodiagnosis of peripheral nerve lesions, *Surg. Gynec. Obstet.*, **81**, 660–6.

Pollock, L. J., Golseth, J. G., Arieff, A. J., Sherman, I. C., Schiller, M. A. and Tigay, E. L. (1944) Electrodiagnosis by means of progressive currents of long duration: studies on cats with experimentally produced section of sciatic nerves, *Arch. Neurol. Psychiat.*, **51**, 147–54.

Pollock, L. J., Golseth, J. G., Arieff, A. J. and Mayfield, F. (1945) Electrodiagnosis by means of progressive currents of long duration, *Surg. Gynec. Obstet.*, **81**, 192–200.

Pollock, L. J., Golseth, J. G., Arieff, A. J., Sherman, I. C., Schiller, M. A. and Tigay, E. L. (1945) Reaction of degeneration in electro-diagnosis of experimental peripheral nerve lesions, *War. Med. (Chic.)*, **7**, 275–83.

Renshaw, B. (1941) Influence of discharge of motoneurons upon excitation of neighbouring motoneurons, *J. Neurophysiol.*, **4**, 167–83.

Richardson, A. T. (1951) Newer concepts of electrodiagnosis, *St Thom. Hosp. Rep.*, **7**, 164–74.

Richardson, A. T. (1956) Clinical and electromyographic aspects of polymyositis, *Proc. roy. Soc. Med.*, **49**, 111–4.

Riecker, G., Dobbelstein, H., Rohl, D. and Bolte, H. D. (1964) Messungen des Membranpotentials einzelner quergestreifter Muskelzellen bei Myotonia congenita, *Thomsen Klin. Wschr.*, **42**, 519–22.

Ritchie, A. E. (1944) The electrical diagnosis of peripheral nerve injury, *Brain*, **67**, 314–30.

Ritchie, A. E. (1948) Thermionic valve stimulators: their value and limitations, *Brit. J. phys. Med.*, **11**, 101–9.

Ritchie, A. E. (1952) Electro-diagnosis—routine or research? *Physiotherapy*, **38**, 151–4.

Ritchie, A. E. (1954) Electrical diagnosis of peripheral nerve injury, in *Periphery Nerve Injuries*. Medical Research Council Special Report Series No. 282. London: HMSO.

Rogoff, J. B. and Reiner, S. (1961) Electrodiagnostic apparatus, in *Electrodiagnosis and Electromyography*. Ed. S. Licht, New Haven, Connecticut: Licht.

Rooke, E. D., Eaton, L. M., Lambert, E. H. and Hodgson, C. J. (1960) Myasthenia and malignant intrathoracic tumour, *Med. Clin. N. Amer.*, **44**, 977–88.

Rose, A. L. and Willison, R. G. (1967) Quantitative electromyography using automatic analysis. Studies in healthy subjects and patients with primary muscle disease, *J. Neurol. Neurosurg. Psychiat.*, **30**, 403–10.

Rushforth, G. (1963) The value and limitations of neurophysiological methods, in *Research in Muscular Dystrophy*, Proc. 2nd Symp.

Current Res. in Muscular Dystrophy, pp. 203–18. London: Pitman Medical.

Sacco, G., Buchthal, F. and Rosenfalck, P. (1962) Motor unit potentials at different ages, *Arch. Neurol. (Chic.)*, **6**, 366–73.

Sanders, F. K. and Whitteridge, D. (1946) Conduction Velocity and myelin thickness in regenerating nerve fibres, *J. Physiol. (Lond.)*, **105**, 152–72.

Sanderson, K. V. and Adey, W. R. (1952) Electromyographic and endocrine studies in chronic thyrotoxic myopathy, *J. Neurol. Neurosurg. Psychiat.*, **15**, 200–5.

Sears, T. A. (1959) Action potentials evoked in digital nerves by stimulation of mechanoreceptors in the human finger, *J. Physiol. (Lond.)*, **148**, 30–1P.

Seddon, H. J. (1943) Three types of nerve injury, *Brain*, **66**, 238–88.

Seyffarth, H. (1941) The behaviour of motor units in healthy and paretic muscles in man, *Acta psychiat. (Kbh.)*, **16**, 79–109, 260–78.

Sherrington, C. S. (1929) Some functional problems attaching to convergence, *Proc. roy. Soc. B*, **105**, 332–62.

Shy, G. M., Engel, W. K., Somers, J. E. and Wanko, T. (1963) Nemaline myopathy; a new congenital myopathy, *Brain*, **86**, 793–810.

Shy, G. M. and Magee, K. R. (1956) A new congenital non-progressive myopathy, *Brain*, **79**, 610–21.

Shy, G. M., Wanko, H., Rowley, P. T. and Engel, A. G. (1961) Studies in familial periodic paralysis, *Exp. Neurol.*, **3**, 53–121.

Silver, I. A. (1958) Other electrodes, in *Electronic Apparatus for Biological Research*, Ed. P. E. K. Donaldson. London: Butterworth.

Simpson, J. A. (1955) On the muscular rigidity and hyperreflexia due to hypothermia in man with observations on the accommodation of peripheral nerve, *J. Neurol. Neurosurg. Psychiat.*, **18**, 191–5.

Simpson, J. A. (1956) Electrical signs in the diagnosis of carpal tunnel and related syndromes, *J. Neurol. Neurosurg. Psychiat.*, **19**, 275–80.

Simpson, J. A. (1960) Myasthenia gravis: a new hypothesis, *Scot. med. J.*, **5**, 419–36.

Simpson, J. A. (1962) Conduction of peripheral nerves in human metabolic disorders, *Electroenceph. clin. Neurophysiol.*, suppl., **22**, 36–43.

Simpson, J. A. (1962) Recent studies of the physiology of the human spinal cord and its disturbance in poliomyelitis, *Proc. 8th Symp. Europ. Ass. Poliomelitis.*, 347–60.

Simpson, J. A. (1964) Fact and fallacy in measurement of conduction velocity in motor nerves, *J. Neurol. Neurosurg. Psychiat.*, **27**, 381–5.

Simpson, J. A. (1966) Control of muscle in health and disease, in *Control and Innervation of Skeletal Muscle.* Ed. B. L. Andrew, 171–80. Edinburgh: E. & S. Livingstone.

Simpson, J. A. (1966) Disorders of neuromuscular transmission, *Proc. roy. Soc. Med.*, **59**, 993–8.

Simpson, J. A., Ed. (1969) Terminology of Electromyography. *Electroenceph. clin. Neurophysiol.*, **26**, 224–6.

Simpson, J. A. and Lenman, J. A. R. (1959) The effect of frequency of stimulation in neuromuscular disease, *Electroenceph. clin. Neurophysiol.*, **11**, 604–5.

Simpson, J. A. (1969) Personal communication.

Sissons, H. A. (1964) The anatomy of the motor unit, in *Disorders of Voluntary Muscle.* Ed. J. N. Walton. London: Churchill.

Slomic, A., Rosenfalck, A. and Buchthal, F. (1968) Electrical and mechanical responses of normal and myasthenic muscle, *Brain Res.*, **10**, 1–78.

Smith, R. and Stern, G. (1967) Myopathy, osteomalacia and hyperparathyroidism, *Brain*, **90**, 593–602.

Solandt, D. Y. (1935) Measurement of human nerve accommodation, *J. Physiol. (Lond.)*, **85**, 5P.

Solandt, D. Y. (1936) Accommodation in nerve, *Proc. roy. Soc. B*, **119**, 355–79.

Spiro, A. J., Shy, G. M. and Gonatas, N. K. (1966) Myotubular myopathy: persistence of fetal muscle in an adolescent boy, *Arch. Neurol. (Chic.)*, **14**, 1–14.

Stephens, W. G. S. (1956) The output impedance of constant-voltage diagnostic stimulators, *Brit. J. phys. Med.*, **19**, 217–23.

Stephens, W. G. S. (1961) A critical survey of the relationship between the output impedance and performance of medical stimulators, *Proc. 3rd int. conf. med. Electronics. Instit. Elect. Eng. London*, 81–6.

Stephens, W. G. S. (1963) The current voltage relationship in the human skin, *Med. Electron. Biol. Engng.*, **1**, 389–99.

Stephens, W. G. S. (1966) The response of human motor nerves to rectangular electric pulses applied through the skin, *Proc. roy. Soc. Edin. B*, **70**, 49–61.

Stephens, W. G. S. (1969) *Proc. roy. Soc. Edin. B*, in press.

Stewart, W. K., Fleming, L. W., Anderson, D. C., Lenman, J. A. R. and Jamieson, D. G. (1968) Changes in plasma electrolytes and nerve-conduction velocities during haemodialysis without magnesium, *Proc. IV E.D.T.A. Conf., Exc. Med. int. Cong. ser.*, **125**, 285–91.

Taverner, D. (1959) The prognosis and treatment of spontaneous facial palsy, *Proc. roy. Soc. Med.*, **52**, 1077–80.

Taverner, D. (1965) Electrodiagnosis in facial palsy, *Arch. Otolaryng.*, **81**, 470–7.

Thage, O. (1965) The 'quadriceps syndrome'. An electromyographic and histological evaluation, *Acta Neurol. scand.*, **41**, suppl. 13, 245–9.

Thesleff, S. (1963) Spontaneous electrical activity in denervated rat skeletal muscle, in *Proc. Symp. on Effect of Use and Disuse on Neuromuscular Functions.* Ed. E. Guttmann, pp. 41–51, Prague: Czech Acad. Sci.

Thom, H. (1953) Elektrotherapis von Lähmungen 'Grundbegriffe und Anwendung, *Ztschr. Orthop.*, **84**, 104–23.

Thomas, J. E. and Lambert, E. H. (1960) Ulnar nerve conduction velocity and H-reflex in infants and children, *J. appl. Physiol.*, **15**, 1–9.

Thomas, P. K. (1960) Motor nerve conduction in the carpal tunnel syndrome, *Neurology (Minneap.)*, **10**, 1045–50.

Thomas, P. K. and Lascelles, R. G. (1965) Schwann-cell abnormalities in diabetic neuropathy, *Lancet*, **i**, 1355–7.

Thomas, P. K. and Morton, H. B. (1963) The electromyographic recording of intensity-duration curves. *Electroenceph. clin. Neurophysiol.*, **15**, 691–8.

Thomas, P. K., Sears, T. A. and Gilliatt, R. W. (1959) The range of conduction velocity in normal motor nerve fibres to the small muscles of the hand and foot, *J. Neurol. Neurosurg. Psychiat.*, **22**, 175–81.

Tokizane, T. and Shimazu, H. (1964) *Functional Differentiation of Human Skeletal Muscle. Corticalization and Spinalization of Movement.* Springfield, Illinois: C. Thomas.

Torre, M. (1953) Nombre et dimensions des unites motrices dans les muscles extrinseques de l'oeil et, en general, dans les muscles squelettiques relies a des organes de sens, *Arch. Suisses Neurol. Psychiat.*, **72**, 362–76.

Trojaborg, W. and Buchthal, F. (1965) Malignant and benign fasciculations, *Acta Neurol. scand.*, **41**, suppl. 13, 251–4.

Van den Bosch, J. (1963) Investigations of the carrier state in muscular dystrophy, in *Research in Muscular Dystrophy*. Proc. 2nd Symp. on Current Res. Muscular Dystrophy, pp. 23–30. London: Pitman Medical.

Wagman, I. H. and Lesse, H. (1952) Maximum conduction velocities of motor fibres of the ulnar nerve in human subjects of various ages and sizes, *J. Neurophysiol.*, **15**, 235–44.

Walker, M. B. (1934) Treatment of myasthenia gravis with physostigmine, *Lancet*, **i**, 1200–1.

Walton, J. N. (1952) The electromyogram in myopathy: analysis with the audio-frequency spectrometer, *J. Neurol. Neurosurg. Psychiat.*, **15**, 219–26.

Walton, J. N. (1963) Progressive muscular dystrophy, in *Disorders of Voluntary Muscle*. Ed. J. N. Walton. London: Churchill.

Walton, J. N. and Adams, R. D. (1958) *Polymyositis*. Edinburgh: E. & S. Livingstone.

Walton, J. N. and Gardner-Medwin, D. (1968) Second thoughts on classification of the muscular dystrophies, in *Research in Muscular Dystrophy*. Proc. 4th Symp. on Current Res. Muscular Dystrophy. pp. 45–71. London: Pitman Medical.

Walton, J. N. and Natrass, F. J. (1954) On the classification, natural history and treatment of the myopathies, *Brain*, **77**, 169–231.

Ware, F., Bennett, A. L. and McIntyre, A. R. (1954) Membrane resting potential of denervated mammalian skeletal muscle measured *in vivo*, *Amer. J. Physiol.*, **177**, 115–18.

Weddell, G., Feinstein, B. and Pattle, R. E. (1944) The electrical activity of voluntary muscle in man under normal and pathological conditions, *Brain*, **67**, 178–257.

Willison, R. G. (1962) Electrodiagnosis in motor neurone disease, *Proc. roy. Soc. Med.*, **55**, 1024–8.

Willison, R. G. (1964) Analysis of electrical activity in healthy and dystrophic muscle in man. *J. Neurol. Neurosurg. Psychiat.*, **27**, 386–94.

Willison, R. G. (1968) The problems of detecting carriers of Duchenne muscular dystrophy by quantitative electromyography, in *Research in Muscular Dystrophy*. Proc. 4th Symp. on Current Res. Muscular Dystrophy, pp. 433–9. London: Pitman Medical.

Wilson, J. and Walton, J. N. (1959) Some muscular manifestations of hypothyroidism, *J. Neurol. Neurosurg. Psychiat.*, **22**, 320–4.

Wohlfart, G. (1958) Collateral regeneration in partially denervated muscles, *Neurology (Minneap.)*, **8**, 175–80.

Wynn Parry, C. B. (1953) Electrical methods in diagnosis and prognosis of peripheral nerve injuries and poliomyelitis, *Brain*, **76**, 229–65.

Wynn Parry, C. B. (1954) The use of electrical methods in the diagnosis and prognosis of peripheral nerve injuries and poliomyelitis. D. M. Thesis, University of Oxford.

Wynn Parry, C. B. (1961) Strength-duration curves, in *Electrodiagnosis and Electromyography*. Ed. S. Licht. New Haven, Connecticut: Licht.

Wynn Parry, C. B. (1961) Electrodiagnosis, *J. Bone Jt. Surg.*, **43B**, 222–36.

Wynn Parry, C. B. (1964) Techniques of neuromuscular stimulation and their clinical application, in *Disorders of Voluntary Muscle*. Ed. J. N. Walton. London: Churchill.

Yap, C-B. (1967) Spinal segmental and long-loop reflexes in spinal motoneurone excitability in spasticity and rigidity, *Brain*, **90**, 887–96.

Index

169